Some Whispers from Eternity

Some Whispers from Eternity

Book on Evolution of Consciousness and Upliftment of Humanity Through OM Kriya Yoga

Shomik Chaudhuri

Motilal Banarsidass Publications

MOTILAL BANARSIDASS
PUBLICATIONS
4741/23, Ansari Road, Daryaganj, New Delhi - 110002 (India)
Email: mlbd@mlbd.com | sales@mlbd.com
exports@mlbd.com | publications@mlbd.com
Website: www.mlbd.com

Some Whispers from Eternity
by
Shomik Chaudhuri

2nd Revised Edition Published in 2025
1st Edition Published in 2023
by Dorrance Publishing Co., USA

South Asian and South East Asian Edition
Published in India by Motilal Banarsidass Publications

ISBN : 978-81-97917-71-4 (PB)

Printed and bound in India

Dedication

The book is dedicated to my revered Adi Guruji, Mahavatar Kriya Babaji, my revered Guruji, Jagadguru Ramanandacharya Rajivlochanacharya and my late parents Barun Kumar Chaudhuri and Swapna Chaudhuri who were all instrumental in helping me be what I am today.

Table of Contents

Introduction

This book was written after seeing and experiencing the total degradation of life on earth, lack of empathy and compassion of humans living here for one another. Humans have created artificial vivisections of the society in every conceivable ways, be it religion, race, caste, creed, region, nation, and so many others. Religious, national strife is a regular feature; humans show hatred toward their fellow beings over nominal things and, of course, the reasons for dissention. The level of consciousness of most people is limited to partying, drinking and making merriment only. There is limited place for self-improvement or inner introspection or self-development. Merriment is good for some time. But the life aims and goals should be understood and practiced and included in people's lifestyle, along with merriment and having a good time.

My understanding, knowledge and experience tells me that human life is the most valuable event to happen to us. We have evolved through innumerous lives to attain the human form. Only the human form has the capability to evolve into the divine state. The aim of our lives is to understand and realize our inner core, which is bliss and divinity. In the book I have enumerated numerous processes that help anyone to practice and evolve into better and more wonderful human beings. These are time tested and authentic processes that make it possible for anyone to practice. A student, a householder, a business- man, a manager, a worker, anyone.

This not only helps you become better but also brings happiness and peace to everything and everyone around you. Studies, work, relationships, experiences all become much better. Concentration, patience, focus, endurance, calm disposition, body fitness among so many others evolve inside you. The quality of life becomes better.

I have learnt, practiced and taught this to many people for over fifty years. I also have had close association with seers who are God-realized and people of great wisdom. Learning from them is a great blessing. But nothing beats the element of practice. Doing sadhana is the best way you can achieve anything and elevate yourself.

The results of this sadhana are too profound and life changing for me. Being an angry young man in my childhood days, I have lost anger in me. I have become more stoic, calm, with tremendous endurance, love and compassion. I am always at peace, meditative and happy. My relationships are now good, my work expresses a much higher quality than before. More than that I do not have any stress, anxiety, worry, and distress at any time.

I also have developed a loving relationship with God and so I always surrender to Him. I have a deep dependence on Him knowing that He will take care of me as long as I do my part. And on innumerous occasions, He does in unbelievable ways.

I can promise that people who read my book and follow the instructions and guidance enumerated there will find an inner transformation within a short time. Along with inner transformation, the outside world will also become more pleasing to you. A life divine and happiness is waiting for you. This is highly secret knowledge and wisdom that has never been distributed and explained in detail before. But Mahavatar Kriya Babaji had instructed my Guruji, Jagadguru Ramanandacharya Rajivlochanacharya, that this wisdom has to reach people globally and without any limitation. So, this wisdom is being shared by me to everyone so that their lives can be fulfilled, and they can lead happy, fulfilled and successful lives. So it is because of his instruction that I share this entire OM Kriya Yoga system with everyone like my revered Guruji did.

I have also worked in my personal capacity with the United Nations through affiliated NGOs. One of them I formed as a cofounder, Institute of International Social Development, based in India, has even received the prestigious Special Consultative Status with ECOSOC of the United Nations for its exemplary work.

I was also selected as the youngest person in UN history to represent the United Nations System in India to the World Summit for Social Development in Copenhagen, Denmark, in March 1995. My paper that I presented in a side event there was that social development starts from the basic level—the human being. A good human being influences the family, the community and the community influences the locality, the locality the region. Many such regions make up a great nation and many such nations build up a better world. I received considerable acclaim for my presentation.

For human beings to be better, they have to better themselves at the physical level, the mental level, the emotional level and the spiritual level. We focus on everything except the spiritual level. But this is the foundation of our very existence. We are spiritual souls and we have to rediscover that through austerities that are explained lucidly and in detail in this book.

Please do not wait for time to pass before you look at this book. Read the book and practice the lessons enumerated there. Life is short. Start today and do not let any day pass by without practicing the lessons and building your relationship with God. Take one step at a time and practice with your sincerity and love for God. He will make your progress faster, easier, and more enjoyable. It should become a part of life and who you are.

I am an ordinary person like everyone. I am not a monk, saint or someone extraordinary. If I can do it, all of you can. So please do your best to practice and evolve yourself to a higher state of existence. There is infinite bliss and a sense of fulfillment in this.

In life we buy, spend and invest in so many things. Most of them are material articles. They are necessary but are not there to help your consciousness to evolve into a higher level of existence. It is not something that can make you prepare for a higher life after death, a better life here, and a better rebirth. Life is a drama. One scene finishes and a new one starts. That is what this life is. As an actor on the stage of life, give your best performance and prepare for the next or prepare to continue living in the higher worlds without ever coming back here.

The choice is yours and the opportunity is here. It is up to you to make the right choice and seek evolution and upliftment in place of stagnation and repeated birth and death cycles.

So, pick up the book and read it and follow it. Such an opportunity seldom comes. Wish you the very best in your path to Godhead.

Foreword

by Parveen Chopra

In his very first book, Some Whispers from Eternity, Shomik Chaudhuri set himself an ambitious and onerous task—to encapsulate the infinitely vast literature of Hinduism in a cogent narrative running into a mere two hundred pages.

Hinduism is not a philosophy or religion. Its correct name is Sanatana Dharma (eternal order), proclaiming that it is a way of life for all human beings at all times and everywhere.

Hinduism is not attributed to a single prophet, like Abraham, Jesus, or Muhammad. Instead, hundreds of Indian sages and yogis dating from millennia ago experimented in the laboratory of life, often on themselves as subjects, to discern, discover and codify the truths that dawned in their consciousness, the eternal laws that govern the cosmic to the human to the atomic levels.

Precisely because Sanatana Dharma is not another religion, the compendium of its knowledge and wisdom with innumerable phalanxes cannot be set in one sacred book like the Torah, Bible, Quran, or Guru Granth Sahib. Our scriptures—Vedas, Shastras, and Puranas—running the gamut of many sciences and streams of life were codified and preserved over centuries in the oral tradition, saved in handwritten manu- scripts, and after Gutenberg they are available in print form.

The spectrum of Vedic knowledge has at one end the most esoteric—Brahman as the ultimate reality, which is both immanent and transcendent.

And at the other end, the secular and practical arts and sciences such as Vedic Mathematics to do even the most complex calculations and calculus in a jiffy; Ayurveda and Yoga as holistic care of body and mind; Jyotish expounding on cosmology, astronomy, and the gravitational pull and effects of large planets on our minds; Vaastu, the science of energy systems in living spaces; and the 64 kalas, or performing arts.

Why is the seemingly mundane and secular considered part and parcel of Vedic scriptures? Because for the Hindu, not just spiritual practices, all human endeavors, all acts, and all actions are to be aimed at self-realization. As Shomik writes in Chapter 6 of his book: "The purpose of life, according to the Vedic tradition, is self-realization and the reestablishment of our lost relationship with the Supreme Being/Godhead."

To keep his narrative lively, Shomik employs an Upanishadic device—the question-and-answer format to dwell on a certain subject and go deep. He starts each of his fifteen chapters with a conversation with his friend Madhu.

Some Whispers from Eternity is not limited to giving a bird's eye view of Vedic literature. In that continuum, Shomik deftly places Kriya Yoga, which has the potential to accelerate your spiritual evolution.

Kriya Yoga is an advanced spiritual system that Paramahansa Yogananda brought to light with his iconic book, *Autobiography of a Yogi*. Shomik learned it as Om Kriya Yoga from his master, Jagadguru Ramanandacharya Rajivlochanacharya, and has practiced it for decades. Shomik, of course, points to Kriya Yoga as a supreme gift from Mahavatar Kriya Babaji, a fabled "Mahamaster," said to be immortal.

Kriya Yoga, Shomik explains, has the concentration factor like other meditation techniques, but makes it more intense with additional kriyas and asanas to enhance the experience of the seeker.

Traditionally, Kriya Yoga lessons are imparted by guru to shishya in an institutional setting, strictly after initiation. Shomik has broken the secrecy around this less-known system and devotes one entire chapter in his book to giving step-by-step Kriya Yoga instructions.

A media person who has had a long association with a United Nations affiliated organization, Shomik concludes by suggesting that the knowledge he has presented should be applied to uplift and transform the entire humanity. After all, the Vedic blessing "Lokah Samastah

Sukhino Bhavantu" is not for Indians only, but for the wellbeing and happiness of all living beings in the world.

As we move slowly but inexorably toward a global Golden Age, thanks to the reemergence of Vedic wisdom and way of life, India would be happy to be deservedly called World Guru.

Parveen Chopra is the founder of ALotusInTheMud.com, a wellness and spirituality web magazine based in New York. He can be reached at editor@alotusinthemud.com.

Chapter 1

The Science of Ancient Vedic Temples

The last rays of the evening sky were streaming onto my sofa from the window in front. I was munching away on some delectable snacks that I had bought from an Indian store in Long Island, New York, snacks on which I had grown up in Kolkata, India. The fall breeze was wafting through the small opening in the windows in my living room. It was the first sign of the forthcoming chill that would envelop most of USA soon. The trembling withered leaves on the trees in the park in front simmered in the breeze and fell in a swoon when the branches could no longer hold them against the pull-and-push of the breeze. It was an otherwise tranquil environment all around except for the sounds of a hungry mouth.

Suddenly the mobile phone rang, breaking the tranquility all around. I checked it with a tinge of pleasure as I found it was my old friend Madhu Sudhan Sharma who was calling. Excited, I picked it up.

"Hi, Madhu, what a pleasant, pleasant surprise. It has been months. Where have you been?" My excitement was unabashed.

"Shomikda,[1] I am so happy to connect with you again. I have just returned a couple of days ago from India. I have been travelling for over six months trekking through the country, checking on its magnificent temples, and

[1] "Da," or "Dada," is a respectful reference to an elder brother, friend or similar relationship in Kolkata.

spiritual destinations from north to south, and east to west. I was thinking of coming and sharing my experiences with you. When will you be free?"

"Tomorrow is Sunday. So why don't you come over for tea at 4 P.M.?" I said.

"That is perfect," he said happily.

I hung up the phone excited at the prospect of meeting Madhu, who is an encyclopedia of knowledge about Indian temples and spiritual destinations.

The next day I sat comfortably on the sofa reading *An Autobiography of a Yogi,* which detailed the metamorphosis of Mukunda to Paramhansa Yogananda. The evening twilight was washing the room with its last golden embers for the day.

I glanced up and saw the clock hand reaching for the 12 o'clock position on the clock to indicate 4 P.M.

I wondered, *I thought Madhu said he will come at 4 P.M. He knows I have great respect for time.*

My thoughts had hardly finished playing themselves out in my mind when the doorbell rang with an all-too-familiar chime and broke the silence in the house.

I got up and went to open the door. There was my friend Madhu with a broad smile exhibiting his near-perfect teeth and exulting in the immense joy that was pouring from his heart.

We embraced each other as he murmured, "Dada, it is so wonderful seeing you after so many months."

"It is so wonderful to see you again, Madhu. Welcome...," I also murmured as I joyfully led him to our living room.

He was about 5'8" height, well built, with a tilak[2] on his forehead, fair but with a dark tan all over from the relentless rays of the sun as he travelled India during the fierce summer months. His face had the calm bliss of a spiritualist and it found further expression through his infectious smile and joyful eyes. He was about forty-five years of age.

As we comfortably settled in our sofas, sitting opposite to each other, my wife presented a plate of freshly baked "samosas"[3] and coffee for our

---

[2] Tilak is the application of sandalwood paste, vermillion, clay or ash in between the eyebrows or on the forehead as a religious practice.

[3] A *samosa* is a fried or baked pastry with a savory filling, such as spiced potatoes, onions, peas, cheese, meats, or lentils.

enjoyment. It was followed by the Indian system of greeting by folding hands and saying "Namaste."[4]

After we had cleared the samosas from the plate, we started the conversation, sipping on the hot coffee.

"So, Madhu, tell me about your journey to India and the experiences that you had," I said at last, not able to withstand the delay any longer.

"Dada," he said, "I started my tour with the world-famous Tirupati[5] temple in South India. Also known as the Venkateshwara Temple, it is situated in the hill town of Tirumala at Tirupati in Chittor district of Andhra Pradesh, India.

"The temple is dedicated to Lord Venkateshwara, a form of Lord Vishnu, and is also known as Balaji, Govinda and Srinivasa.

"The construction of the temple, built in the unique architecture seen in temples in the South of India, is believed to have started around 300 A.D. The Sanctum Sanctorum is called Ananda Nilayam. The presiding deity Venkateshwara is in a standing posture and faces east. It is one of the eight Vishnu Swayambhu Khetras[6] and is listed as 106th and the last earthly Divya

Desam.[7] "It is the richest temple in the world in terms of donations and wealth that it has. The initial wealth of the temple owed its origin to the Pallava, Chola and Vijayanagar empires, who were devotees of Lord Venkateshwara.

"Garbhagriha is the Sanctum sanctorum where presiding deity Lord Venkateshwara resides along with other deities. A golden entrance leads to the garbhagriha. The deity is standing with four hands, one in a veranda or blessing posture, one placed over the thighs, one holding the Shankha or conch shell and the other holding the Sudarshana Chakra. [8] The deity is decorated with precious ornaments. The deity bears Goddess Lakshmi on the right chest and Goddess Padmavathi on the left.

"Ananda Nilayam Vimanam is the main three-storied Gopuram[9] constructed above the Sanctum sanctorum. It is covered with gilt copper plates

---

[4] The ancient Hindu practice is a way of greeting and saying "I bow to the divinity in you."

[5] Source: *www.tirumala.org.*

[6] There are eight self-manifested temples of Lord Vishnu. It is believed that Lord Vishnu appeared here and the main deity worshipped here is of divine origin.

[7] Divya Desam means one of the 108 temples, or "divine abodes," of Lord Vishnu that are mentioned in the works of saints.

[8] Sudarshana Chakra is a spinning-wheel weapon, having 108 serrated edges used by Lord Vishnu. It means "auspicious vision."

[9] Gopuram is a monumental entrance tower, usually ornate, at the entrance of a Hindu temple in South India.

and covered with a gold vase. There are many deities carved over the Gopuram. On this Gopuram, there is a deity of Lord Venkateshwara known as 'Vimana Venkateshwara.'

"Another important aspect of the temple visit is circumambulation around the Sanctum sanctorum of the temple or deity and is also very important, called Pradakshinam. There are two circumambulation paths in the temple. The first one is the area between *Mahaprakaram* and *Sampangiprakaram*. This path, known as *Sampangipradakshinam*, has many Mandapas, Dwajasthambam, Balipeetam, Kshetrapalika sila, and prasadam distribution area, among other areas. The *Vimanapradakhinam* is the second *pradakshinam*, which circumbulates *Ananda Nilayam Vimanam*. This path has sub-shrines dedicated to Varadaraja and Yoga Narasimha, Potu (main kitchen), Bangaru Bavi (golden well), Ankurarpana Mandapam, Yagasala, Nanala (coins and Notla (paper notes)) Parkamani, Almyrah of Sandal paste (Chandanapu ara), cell of records, Sannidhi Bhashyakarulu, Lord's hundi and the seat of Vishvaksena. I took the first one and had a most elevating experience.

"Getting a darshan or divine view of the Lord can be done through the regular way where you have to stand in the line for hours or else you buy a special ticket and get the darshan in a very short time. I chose the latter and as I wound my way to the inner sanctum, I felt the deep divine vibration there and a tremendous peace descended on me during my time at the inner sanctum. I will never forget it in my life. I left with the famous [10]Laddu Prasad as an additional reward."

After this long lecture, Madhu stopped to take a few sips of his coffee. I asked him, "Do you know the science behind the construction of the Vedic temples in ancient time?"

Madhu looked at me a little puzzled and quizzed, "What is the science behind these extraordinary constructions?"

I took a sip of a new cup of hot coffee that my dear wife had just prepared and replied to Madhu. [11]"In the Vedic times and culture, the temple was seen as a link between man and God, and between the actual and the ultimate. As such it has got to be symbolic. A temple usually called Devalaya, the abode of God, is also referred to as Prasada, meaning a palace with very pleasing aspects. Vimana is another term that denotes

---

[10] Special sweetmeat given to pilgrims in Tirupati is called Tirupati Laddu.

[11] Source: *https://www.sanskritimagazine.com.*

temple in general and the Sanctum and its dome, in particular. Thirtha, a place of pilgrimage, is its other name. The entire construction is based on the science of Vastu. The science of Vastu is believed as part of the Indian architecture from the ancient times. Vastu Shastra is supposed to have developed during the period of 6000 B.C. and 3000 B.C. and the ancient Indian text Mayamatam represents Vastu Purusha as the presiding deity for all land structure meant for temples or houses. Vastu Purusha Mandala is the metaphysical plan of a temple incorporating course of the heavenly bodies and supernatural forces. This Mandala square is divided into (8×8 =64) 64 metaphysical grids / modules or pada for temples.

"The Vastu Purusha Mandala represents the manifest form of the Cosmic Being, upon which the temple is built and in whom the temple rests. The temple is situated in Him, comes from Him, and is a manifestation of Him. The Vastu Purusha Mandala is both the body of the Cosmic Being and a bodily device by which those who have the requisite knowledge attain the best results in temple building (Stella Kramrisch, The Hindu Temple, Vol. I).

"The Vastu Purusha is pictured as lying with his face and stomach on the ground to suggest he is carrying the weight of the structure. His head is at northeast (ishanya) and his legs are at the southwest corner (nairutya).

"The southwest corner (nairutya), where the Vastu Purusha has his legs, corresponds to the Muladhara chakra and denotes the earth principle.

"As the legs support the weight of the body, the base (adhistana) for the muladhara should be steady and strong. Accordingly, the southwest portion of the building is the loadbearing area and should be strong enough to support heavy weights. As the feet are warm, the southwest cell represents warmth and heat; even according to the atmospheric cycles the southwest region receives comparatively more heat.

"Svadhistana chakra is in the lower stomach region near the kidneys. It is related to the water principle (apa). On the Vastu Purusha Mandala it is to the south and to the west. Therefore, wet areas like bathroom and other areas dealing with water, are suggested in the south or in the west portions of the building. It is for sewerage (utsarjana).

"Manipura Chakra is at the navel and relates to energy or fire or tejas. While in the womb of the mother, the baby is fed with the essence of food and energy through the umbilical cord connected with its navel. The Vastu

Purusha Mandala shows Brahman at the navel of the Vastu Purusha. Further, the lotus is the base (Adhistana) of Brahman. Thus, navel connects Brahman with Jiva or life. It is left open and unoccupied. The central portion of the building is to be kept open. It is believed that Vastu Purusha breathes through this open area.

"Anahata chakra is near the heart. It is related to vayu or air regulated by lungs. The lung region of the Vastu Purusha should have more air. Vishuddaha chakra is near the throat, from where the sounds come out and reverberate in space. This region represents space (akasha).The primordial word OM is chanted through the throat. The echo of that sound vibrates in the hollow of the bone-box of the head and in the space in brain. The head of Vastu Purusha is at the northeast corner (Ishanya). The Ajna chakra is between the eyebrows. This direction is related to open spaces (akasha). Atmospherically, northeast is cooler and so should be one's head. The puja room Devagraha is recommended in the northeast portion of the house. The limbs of Vastu Purusha, other than the above, are also associated with the construction of the building. Liver (yakrt) is toward southeast. The cooking area is recommended in south- east, because it is related to Agni. The rays of sun reach here first and cleanse the atmosphere.

"The northwest, vayuvya, is presided over by air vayu. The organs like spleen, rectum of the Vastu Purusha fall in this portion. The storeroom is recommended here, perhaps because the spleen in the body does the work of storing and restoring blood. Directions in Hindu tradition are called as Disa, or Dik. There are four primary directions and a total of ten directions: east, southeast (Agneya), west, northwest (Vayavya), north, northeast (Isanya), south, southeast (Nauritya), Zenith (Urdhva), and Nadir (Adho). There are 'Guardians of the Directions' (Dikpala, or Dasa-dikpala) who rule the exact directions of space.

"So, this is the science behind the construction of the ancient Vedic temples, which were powerhouses of enormous positive energy in tune with the vibrations of the cosmos, which brought about a lot of upliftment in the people who visited them."

Madhu was a silent but focused listener to my talk on the science behind the construction of Vedic temples in ancient times. Except for frequent sips of coffee, his eyes were glued to mine and he was drinking every word that emanated from me.

At last, he spoke. "So, Shomikda, science was very much advanced in ancient India that can even challenge modern scientists?"

"Yes," I said with a smile, "we have forgotten our heritage under the barrage of negative forces, impositions and false narratives. But even today, the architecture of the Hindu temples of mainly South India bear witness to our brilliance in technology and science that are etched in the carvings on the hardest stones that can be found on earth. It will more than challenge today's sculptors too. We need to rediscover our heritage, wisdom and culture as it is geared to help entire humanity, the environment and Nature and not be limiting to one's own selfish benefits at the cost of the destruction of everyone and everything else."

It was late in the evening. The rustling of the falling leaves in the waft of the gentle breeze gained more prominence as we fell silent. Madhu and I were engrossed in getting an understanding of what discussion transpired between us for the past few hours.

"What an evening, Shomikda!" Madhu finally exclaimed, coming out of his stupor. "Let us meet soon. I have so many more temples to talk about. My experience with these visits is mindboggling. How about next weekend?"

I nodded in appreciation and acceptance.

My wife and I saw him to the door with the last-minute Indian habit of elongated goodbyes at the door. I saw him drive off into the evening as the golden rays of the setting sun bathed the Long Island town as it bid goodbye also for the night.

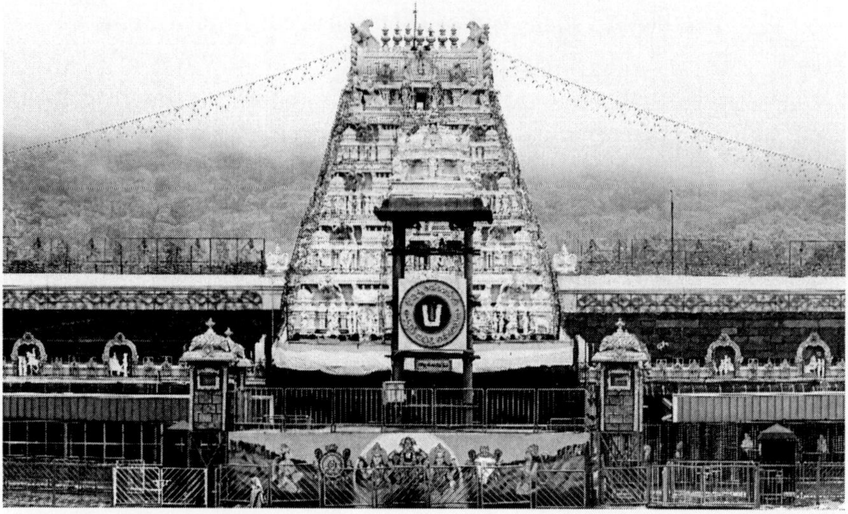

Misty morning at the Tirupati Temple. Credit: Krishna Narendra

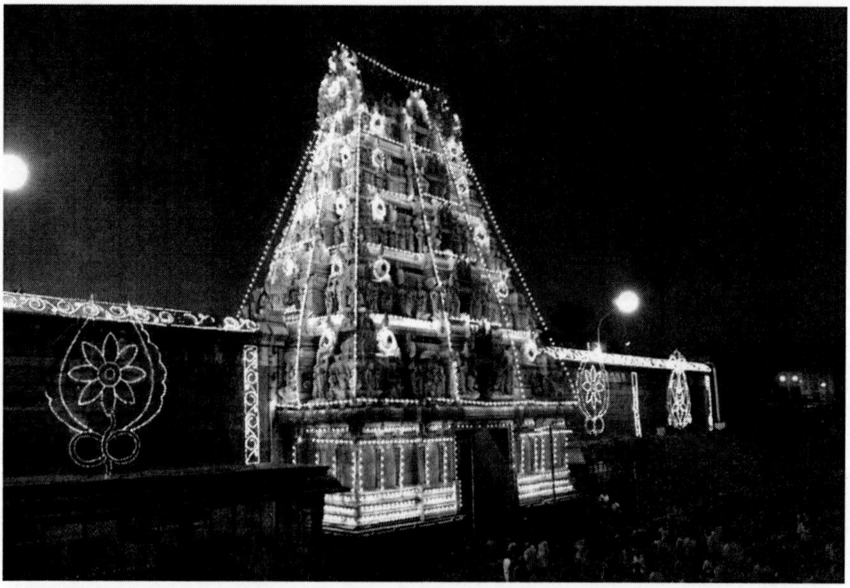

Night View of Tirupati Temple. Credit: Ministry of External Affairs, Government of India

Chapter 2
The Koshas

Madhu called me a few days after our last meeting when I was in the middle of a meeting in the early afternoon of a beautiful fall day. Gorgeous, pleasant rays of the sun streamed in from the glass window that was partially covered by a thick drape.

"Shomikda, could we meet over the weekend?" he asked, sounding excited.

I asked him, "Sure, anything exciting? You seem to be very excited about something."

"Yes, Shomikda. I wanted to know more about our existence, the science of our very beings. And I want to share about the beautiful temples that I have been touring for so long in India. Can we meet this Saturday at a Starbucks coffee shop?" he asked, seemingly pleading for a confirmation.

"Yes," I said, "let us meet in the Starbucks coffee shop in Lynbrook. At 4 P.M. this Saturday."

The Saturday afternoon was bathed in pleasant sunshine, with a cool fall breeze flowing through our bodies as Madhu and I strolled toward the Starbucks shop. The sitting places were nearly full, except two for us, which suited us perfectly. After ordering two lattes, we settled down at the small table that we had and smiled at each other.

"Shomikda, can you please explain the science behind our very existence? I am so eager to know more about the science after your illuminating talk about the science of the Vedic architecture last time. It is amazing," he said with suppressed excitement.

It is always pleasing to share your knowledge with someone as curious and hungry for wisdom as Madhu.

I started talking while sipping on my latte. "The human being is made up of several layers of bodies that make up our human existence.

"Annamaya Kosha (Physical Sheath)[12]

[13]"From the Atma or soul, space is born; from Akasa or space, air; from air, fire; from fire, water; from water, fire; from earth, herbs; from herbs, food; and from food, man. Though the physical sheath, or physical body, is the most tangible aspect of ourselves, very few of us have a real sense of where our organs are or what goes on inside our bodies. When we eat any food, we eat it due to the appearance, the smell and, of course, the taste. However, we do not try to understand how it will react once it goes to the inside of our bodies. We do not feel our bodies inside and feel the numerous processes going on inside the body for our lifetimes. If we really focus on our inside bodies, then we will get an idea as to what is good for the body and what is not. Once you learn to feel your body, to sense it from within, you will learn how to sense what kind of food you need and how much. Your attention will become grounded. Consciously inhabiting your physical body will bring more presence and ease to your life.

"Using this kosha: To get into the physical body, try this exercise. Notice your feet in your shoes. Tighten and relax the muscles in your calves. Touch your face and sense the contact between the fingers and the skin. Put your hand over your chest and feel your heartbeat or feel the contact between the hand and the flesh. Then pick an inner organ—your liver, heart, or kidneys—and try to find it with your attention. Really sink your attention into that organ. Notice the settling and grounding effect of this practice.

"Pranamaya Kosha (Vital Energy Sheath)

"The next three *koshas* are subtle—they can't be tangibly grasped. Nonetheless, they can be felt and feeling them is essential for mastery of your inner world.

"The *pranamaya kosha*, or vital energy body, interpenetrates the physical body but is much larger. [14]When you feel energy expanding into your heart or

---

[12] *https://www.yogajournal.com/Yoga-101/philosophy/getting-know/.*

[13] Taittriya Upanishad.

[14] There are pancha (five) pranas: Prana, Apana, Vyana, Udana, Samana. The sum total of energy is called "Cosmic Prana."

head during meditation or asana practice, or when waves of heat ripple through your body, you are in contact with the vital energy body. Having the feeling of being energized, sleepy, dull, restless, or calm are all attributes of the vital energy body. Just as you have a physical 'look,' you also have a personal energetic body. Once you become sensitive to the energy within and around you, you will start to recognize the vibrational frequency that you and others leave in a room, or even on a piece of clothing.

"You may also notice how much of your communication with the world happens on an energetic level. Imagine the way you feel when you're in a congregation of materialistic people making useless talk, the peace you can find by sitting under a shady tree, the subtle transmission of energy you get from being near a self-realized saint.

"Meditation is a tool that we use to become meditative. It is intended to tone the energy body, as is asana practice. We often think of these practices as toning the mental and physical bodies, respectively, but Yoga and meditation are also aimed at moving stagnant energy, or *prana*, through the body. One way to tune in to the power within the energy body is to practice letting yourself 'be breathed.' Without changing your breathing pattern, become aware of the breath flowing into and out of your body as a natural, spontaneous flow.

"Using this kosha: Notice your breathing. If you notice your breath tightening, just notice it, with the thought 'I am being breathed.' Eventually you may begin to feel the breath as energy, and you may sense that the body is bigger than the boundaries of the skin. This is a sign that you've entered the vital energy body. Now you are consciously accessing the vital energy body, which is the storehouse of healing power in your system.

"Manomaya Kosha (Mental Body)

"The *manomaya kosha*—within which you think, fantasize, daydream, and practice mantra or affirmations—is the part of you that creates meaning out of the world you inhabit. But just as the physical body has layers of skin, fat, blood, and bones, so the mental body has its own layers. The most superficial layer comprises passing thoughts, images, perceptions, and emotions that come up in your inner world.

"However, if some of the thoughts in the *manomaya kosha* are like bubbles in the ocean, others are like tides and have a stronger hold. The deeper levels of the *manomaya kosha* contain the powerful mental structures formed by the beliefs, opinions, and assumptions that you've absorbed from your family and culture as well as from your accumulated mental patterns. Called *samskaras* in Sanskrit, these deep thought grooves in the mental body cause your perceptions of yourself and your life to run in certain fixed patterns. When you examine the contents of the *manomaya kosha* closely, you can often see these patterns, which take the form of repetitive. *Samskaras* not only color your experience but also help shape it.

"Using this kosha: Use this basic self-inquiry, adapted from an exercise developed by the spiritual teacher Byron Katie. Check out a situation in your life that is charged in some way. Write down your thoughts about it. Then, one by one, consider each thought and ask yourself, 'What would I be without this thought?' Check how you're breathing, your energy, and your mental experience shift.

"Consciously swap the thought with one that feels enabling and real—such as 'I am free to choose my attitudes' or 'There are other possibilities to see this.' Notice whether this new thought brings greater capaciousness to your mind.

"Vijnanamaya Kosha (Wisdom or Awareness Body)

"As you explore your inner world, you may begin to notice that along with your thoughts there are things that come from a deeper and subtler level of your being. This sense of inner knowledge comes from the wisdom body, the layer composed of intuition and awareness. The wisdom body is also responsible for insight. If you become engrossed in a project like writing, painting, mathematics, or even finding solutions to problems, you're accessing the wisdom body.

"A composer often plays random music until his regular mind (his *manomaya kosha*) steps back, enabling for the wisdom body to 'download' music that is genuinely creative and new. Another person said that when he's stymied or trapped on a personal or professional problem, he'll frame a question about it, then sit for meditation. At some point, as his thinking mind gets quiet, wisdom will arise. The wisdom body, at its subtlest level, is just awareness—the objective, observing part of the self. It's where you can stop identifying with your powerful thoughts and self-descriptions, and just witness your mind and your life.

"Using this kosha: Right now, notice that something in you witnesses that you are reading. That same witnessing 'I' is also aware of your thoughts, your mood, the way your body feels, your energy level. It knows all this without being involved in it. As you embody awareness, notice if you are able to contain all the other levels of experience—without getting attached to their meaning or outcome.

"Anandamaya Kosha (Bliss Body)

"The bliss body is the most hidden part of us, yet its subtle presence is felt as the instinctive sense that life is worth living, that it is good to be alive. You're literally born to be blissful, because the bliss body is the deepest layer of your personal Self. Separated by a thread from the universal Self, your bliss body is filled with natural ecstasy, vitality, and goodness.

"Connection with the bliss body develops through practice of mantra, meditation, and prayer that teach the mind to let go of the thoughts that hide the bliss body. To fully move in to the bliss body, however, you usually need to be in a state of deep meditation. When you are in touch with your bliss body, you know that your nature is blissful, free, and capable of every flavor of happiness from absolute ecstasy to just contentment. You are in the bliss body in those moments during which you recognize—viscerally rather than intellectually—that love is the deepest reality, beyond mental concepts or ideas. In fact, one of Yoga's greatest reward is its power to awaken us to our body of bliss.

"Using this kosha: Ask yourself, 'Where is bliss?' Ask in an open-ended way and tune in to the subtle feelings of tenderness, bliss, and satisfaction that can show up at the most unexpected of moments. Understand that bliss is your true nature. Don't worry if there is no immediate answer or response. The bliss body takes time to reveal itself. For many sadhakas, the experience of the bliss body arises after years of dedicated practice. Yet it can come alive for you in a moment—during an evening of devotional music or a meditation on the heart, or in deep Savasana (Corpse Pose). When the bliss body does reveal itself, it can seem miraculous, like a gift, and yet completely natural. Your essence is innately blissful. But you need to learn and practice to turn deep inside to recognize it."

I added, "There is also the 'True Essence' of Human Existence, which are the changeless, eternal witness, the uncreated, unmanifested Primordial Nature, Intelligence, the Ego, Self-consciousness, Mind, the five sense-organs for Hearing, Feeling by Touch, Seeing, Tasting, Smelling, the five motor-organs for Speaking, Grasping, Moving, Excreting, Sexual Activities, the five subtle elements—Sound, Touch, Color, Flavor and Odor—and the five gross elements—Ether, Air, Fire, Water and Earth.

"We are all part of this Existence. Initially, the Lord was all alone. He desired to become many and be born. He performed austerities and created this Creation that we see. Having created it, He entered into it. Having entered it, He became the manifest and the unmanifest, the defined and the undefined, the housed and the houseless, knowledge and ignorance, truth and falsehood, and all this whatsoever that exists. That is why it is called Existence."

Our lattes had cooled down considerably from the steaming versions as we were engrossed in discussion on these subjects.

"Shomikda, there is so much for us to learn about ourselves about which we have limited or no idea," Madhu finally broke the silence as we were sipping our lattes unconsciously, delving on the subject of discussion intently.

"Madhu, tell me about more temples that you have visited," I finally appealed to him.

"Shomikda, I went to the Meenakshi Temple in the town of Madurai in Tamil Nadu. [15]Meenakshi Amman Temple, also known as Meenakshi-Sundareshwara Temple, is one of the oldest and most important temples in India. Located in the city of Madurai, the temple has great mythological and historical significance. It is believed that Lord Shiva assumed the form of Sundareswarar (the handsome one) and married Parvati (Meenakshi) at the site where the temple is currently located. Renowned for its astonishing architecture, Meenakshi Temple was nominated as one of the wonders of the world but couldn't make it into the list of 'Seven Wonders of the World.' However, the temple is definitely one of the 'Wonders of India.' It is also one of the main attractions of South India with thousands of devotees thronging it every day. During the 'Tirukalyanam Festival,' which takes place over a period of ten days, the temple attracts more than a million devotees. Despite many people visiting it every day, the temple is well-maintained and was named the 'Best Swachh Iconic Place' (cleanest iconic place) in India.

---

[15] *https://www.culturalindia.net/indian-temples/meenakshi-temple.html.*

"Mythology

"According to a legend, Meenakshi emerged out of a 'Yajna' (sacred fire) as a three-year-old girl. The 'Yajna' was performed by a king named Malayadwaja Pandya, along with his wife, Kanchanamalai. Since the royal couple had no child, the king offered his prayers to Lord Shiva, requesting him to grant them a son. But to their dismay, a triple-breasted girl emerged from the sacred fire. When Malayadwaja and his wife expressed their concern over the girl's abnormal appearance, a divine voice ordered them not to fret over the girl's physical appearance. They were also informed that the girl's third breast would disappear as soon as she met her future husband. The relieved king named her Meenakshi and in due course crowned her as his successor.

"Meenakshi ruled over the ancient city of Madurai and also went on to capture the neighboring kingdoms. Legend has it that she even captured Indralok, the abode of Lord Indra, and was on her way to capture Kailash, the abode of Lord Shiva, as well. When Shiva appeared before her, Meenakshi's third breast disappeared and she knew that she had met her better half. Shiva and Meenakshi returned to Madurai, where their wedding took place. It is said that the wedding was attended by all the gods and goddesses. Since Parvati herself had assumed the form of Meenakshi, Lord Vishnu, Parvati's brother, handed her over to Lord Shiva. Even today, the wedding ceremony is celebrated every year as 'Chithirai Thiruvizha,' which is also known as 'Tirukalyanam' (the grand wedding).

"History

"The history of Meenakshi Temple dates back to the 1st century C.E., with scholars claiming it to be as old as the city itself. It is said that Kulashekarar Pandyan, a king who ruled over the Pandyan dynasty, built the temple as per the instructions given in his dream by Lord Shiva. A few religious texts that belong to the 1st to 4th century C.E. talk about the temple and describe it as the central structure of the city. Texts dating back to the early 6th century describe the temple as a place where scholars met to discuss important topics. The temple as it stands today, however, was rebuilt throughout the 16th century as it was destroyed by the Muslim invaders.

"During the 14th century C.E., Malik Kafur, a commander of Delhi Sultanate, led his army into most parts of Southern India and looted many temples, including the famed Meenakshi Temple. Valuables such as gold, silver and precious gems were taken to Delhi. Since temples in those days had abundance of valuables, most of the temples were destroyed and were left in ruins. When the Vijayanagar Empire took over Madurai after defeating the Muslim Sultanate, the temple was rebuilt and reopened. The temple was further expanded during the late 16th century and early 17th century by Vishwanatha Nayakar, a king of the Nayaka dynasty. According to researchers, while rebuilding the temple, the rulers of Nayaka dynasty followed the architectural style of 'Silpa Shastras.' 'Silpa Shastras' are a set of architectural laws found in ancient texts.

"The temple was once again expanded by Thirumalai Nayak, who ruled over Madurai from 1623 to 1655. During his reign, many 'Mandapams' (pillared halls) were built. The temple was then expanded by many later Nayaka rulers before the advent of the British East India Company. The temple was once again degraded and parts of it were destroyed during the British Rule. In 1959, the restoration work was started by Tamil Hindus by collecting donations and by collaborating with historians and engineers. The temple was completely restored in 1995.

"Temple Structure

"The temple occupies a huge area in the heart of Madurai as it spreads over fourteen acres. The temple is enclosed with huge walls, which were built in response to the invasions. The entire structure, when viewed from above, represents a mandala. A mandala is a structure built according to the laws of symmetry and loci. There are various shrines built within the temple complex. Apart from the two main shrines, which are dedicated to Sundareswarar and Meenakshi, the temple has shrines dedicated to various other deities like Ganesha and Murugan. The temple also houses goddesses Lakshmi, Rukmini, and Saraswati.

"The temple also has a consecrated pond named 'Porthamarai Kulam.' The term 'Porthamarai Kulam' is a literal translation of 'pond with a golden lotus.' The structure of a golden lotus is placed at the center of the pond. It is said that Lord Shiva blessed this pond and declared that no marine life would grow in it. In the Tamil folklore, the pond is believed to be an evaluator for reviewing the worth of any new literature.

"The temple has four main towering gateways (gopurams) that look identical to each other. Apart from the four 'gopurams,' the temple also houses many other 'gopurams' that serve as gateways to number of shrines. The temple has a total of fourteen towering gateways. Each one of them is a multi-story structure and displays thousands of mythological stories and several other sculptures. The major 'gopurams' of the temple are:

Kadaka Gopuram-This towering gateway leads to the main shrine that houses Goddess Meenakshi. The gateway was rebuilt by Tumpichi Nayakkar during the mid-16th century. The 'gopuram' has five stories.

Sundareswarar Shrine Gopuram -This is the oldest 'gopuram' of the temple and was built by Kulasekara Pandya. The 'gopuram' serves as a gateway to the Sundareswarar (Lord Shiva) shrine.

Chitra Gopuram -Built by Maravarman Sundara Pandyan II, the gopuram depicts the religious and secular essence of Hinduism.

Nadukkattu Gopuram -Also called as the 'Idaikattu Gopuram,' this gateway leads to the Ganesha shrine. The gateway is placed right in between the two main shrines.

Mottai Gopuram - This 'gopuram' has fewer stucco images when compared to the other gateways. Interestingly, 'Mottai gopuram' had no roof for nearly three centuries.

Nayaka Gopuram -This 'gopuram' was built by Visvappa Nayakkar around 1530. The 'gopuram' is astonishingly similar to another gateway called 'Palahai Gopuram.'

"The temple also has numerous pillared halls called 'Mandapams.' These halls were built by various kings and emperors and they serve as resting places for pilgrims and devotees. Some of the most important 'mandapams' are:

Ayirakkal Mandapam -It literally translates to 'hall with thousand pillars.' The hall, which was built by Ariyanatha Mudaliar, is a true spectacle as it is supported by 985 pillars. Each and every pillar is sculpted magnificently and has images of Yali, a mythological creature.

Kilikoondu Mandapam -This 'mandapam' was originally built to house hundreds of parrots. The parrots that were kept there in cages were trained to say 'Meenakshi.' The hall, which is next to the Meenakshi shrine, has sculptures of characters from Mahabharata.

Ashta Shakthi Mandapam -This hall houses the sculptures of eight goddesses. Built by two queens, the hall is placed in between the main 'gopuram' and the gateway that leads to the Meenakshi shrine.

Nayaka Mandapam –'Nayaka Mandapam' was built by Chinnappa Nayakkar. The hall is supported by one hundred pillars and houses a Nataraja statue.

"Significance and Worship

"Since Meenakshi is the main deity of the temple, the temple signifies the importance of woman in a Tamil Hindu family. The temple also portrays the cordial relationship between Shaivism, Vaishnavism and Shaktism. The Sundareswarar shrine is known as one-fifth of 'Pancha Sabhai' (five courts), where Lord Shiva is believed to have performed the cosmic dance. Worship mainly involves rituals and processions. One of the rituals involves placing an image of Sundareswarar inside a palanquin, which is then moved to the shrine of Meenakshi. The palanquin is taken into the shrine every night and is brought back to the shrine of Sundareswarar every morning. The devotees usually worship Meenakshi before offering their prayers to Sundareswarar.

"Festivals

"Apart from the main festival, which is basically the wedding ceremony of the deities, a number of other festivals are celebrated in the temple. Some of these include 'Vasantham festival,' 'Unjal festival,' 'Mulai-Kottu festival,' 'Arudhra Darshan festival,' 'Thai utsavam,' 'Kolattam festival,' etc. Each of these festivals has its own significance and is celebrated during various months throughout the year. The temple also celebrates 'Navarathri festival.' During 'Navarathri' the temple displays colorful dolls, which are collectively called 'gollu.' 'Gollu' often convey stories from mythological scenes."

Madhu took a break and finished his latte in a quick gulp and looked at me with interest. What was my reaction to his experiences?

"Madhu, you are very fortunate to visit the ancient temple cities of India, where our ancestors knew how to energize through scientific consecration. Such sciences were more common before the invading barbarians burnt down thirteen ancient universities and destroyed all the manuscripts containing all the sciences.

"Let us meet again for further discussion about the temples of India and our human existence. See you tomorrow," I said with an air of deep satisfaction.

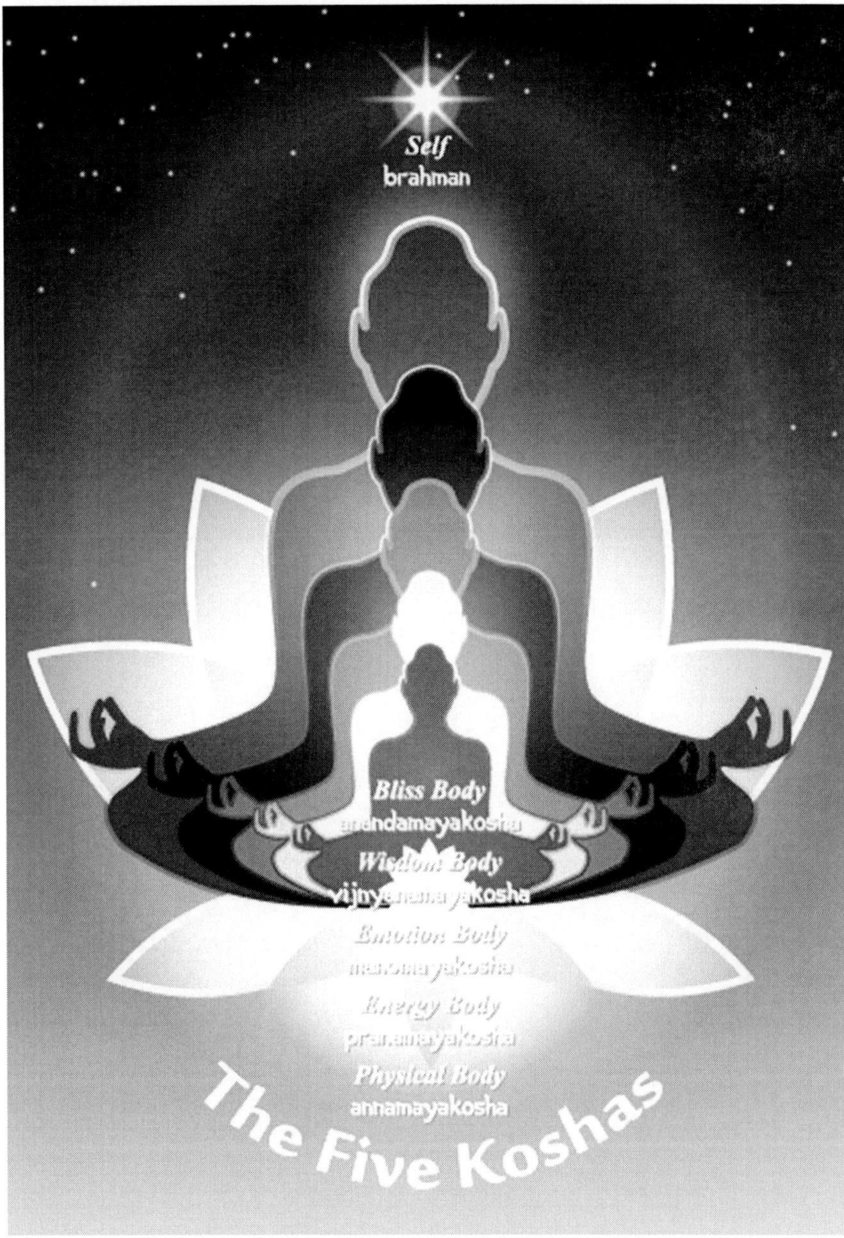

Creative representation of the five energy subtle bodies of man as a covering of the Atma. Credit: Sergey7777

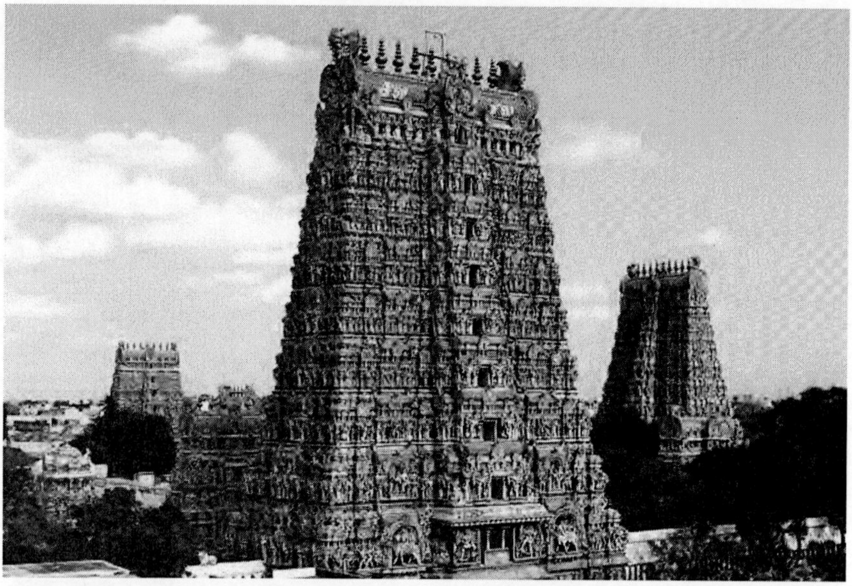

Meenakshi Sundareswarar Temple in Madurai, Tamil Nadu, India. It is a twin temple, one of which is dedicated to Meenakshi, and the other to Lord Sundareswarar. Credit: Rafal Cichawa

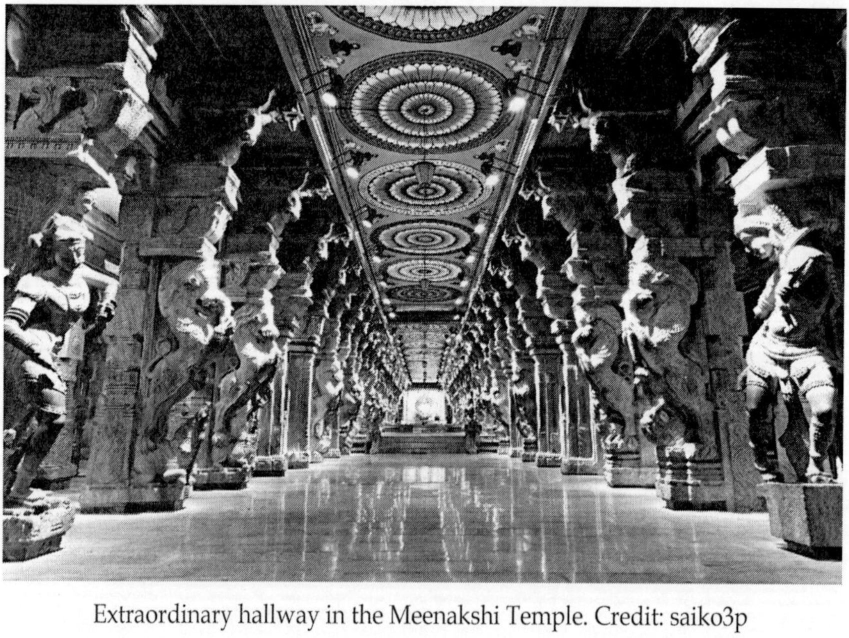

Extraordinary hallway in the Meenakshi Temple. Credit: saiko3p

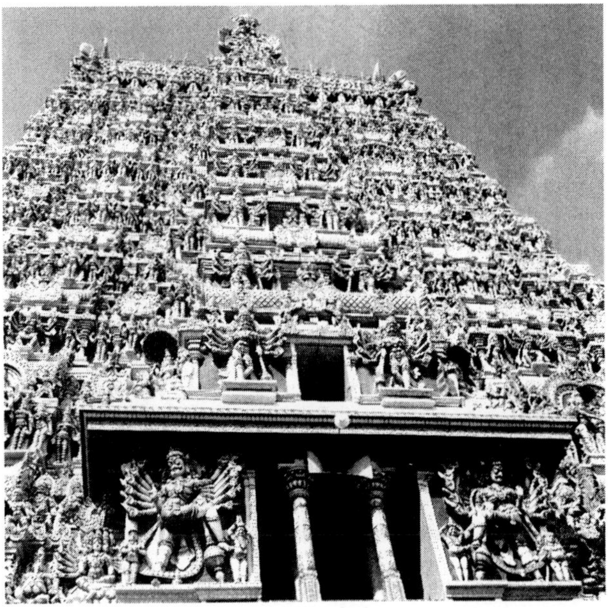

View of Meenakshi Temple. Credit: Ministry of External Affairs, Government of India

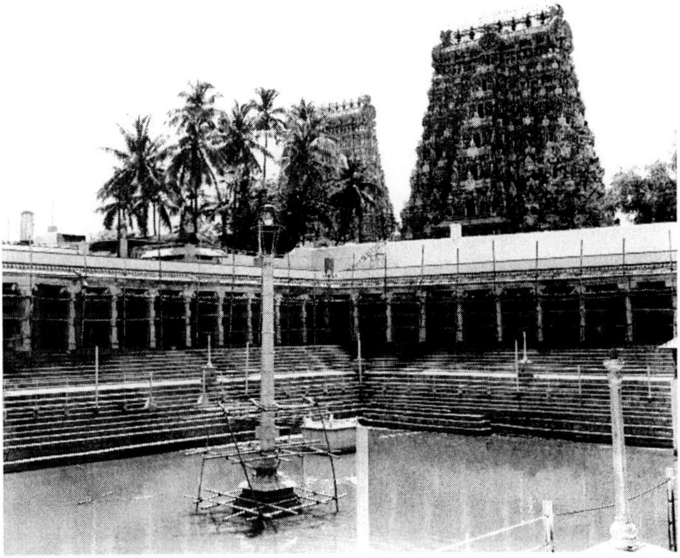

View of Meenakshi Temple. Credit: Ministry of External Affairs, Government of India

Chapter 3
The Chakras

The next day, being a Sunday, Madhu invited me to come to his home, a small apartment in Forest Hills in the Queens borough of New York City. Being a bachelor, he is happy with his studio apartment with quaint furniture and yet having a glowing set of photos of the deities that he had visited in the temples of India over the years. There was peace and serenity in his beautiful apartment.

I had a glass of orange juice handed over to me with cookies on the table in front of us. Excellent for starting a conversation.

"Today let me talk about chakras, which hold your body's energy (or *prana*) and your actions can help keep it in balance,"[16] I started.

"The Sanskrit word 'chakra' refers to a wheel or disk. In Yoga, meditation, and Ayurveda, this term refers to wheels of energy throughout the body. There are seven main chakras that align along the spine, starting from the base of the spine to the crown of the head. The spheres run along the spine, but extend through and past the front, back, and both sides of your body. *Chakras* are spinning whirlpools of energy that are not seen by the human eye but can be seen, felt, and sensed with intuition. This invisible healing energy, called prana, is a vital life force, which keeps us vibrant, healthy, and alive.

"*Chakras* store the energy of thoughts, feelings, memories, experiences, and actions. They affect and direct our present and future attitude, behavior, emotional health, and actions. The life force in each chakra can be treated,

---

[16] *Chopra.com.*

transformed and released so that we willfully manifest what we want to call in, rather than experience more of the same. *Chakra* healing is the willful practice of connecting with our stored energy, so we may understand how our past is influencing the present and the future. *Prana* tells us, and impacts our actions and behaviors, shaping our health, career prospects, relationships, and more. The subtle body shows how our inner reality creates our outer reality.

"These spinning wheels of energy correspond to huge nerve centers in the body. Each of the seven main *chakras* contain bundles of nerves and major organs as well as our psychological, emotional, and spiritual states of being. Since everything is moving, it's essential that our seven main *chakras* stay open, aligned, and fluid. If there is a blockage, energy flows are restricted. Think of something as simple as your washbasin drain. If you allow too much hair to go into the drain, the washbasin will back up with water, stagnate, and eventually bacteria and mold will grow. So, it is too with our bodies and the *chakras*. A washbasin is simple; it's physical so the fix is easy. Keeping a chakra open is a bit more of a challenge, but not so difficult when you have awareness. Since mind, body, soul, and spirit are closely connected, awareness of an imbalance in one area through chakra meditation will help bring the others back into balance. Take, for example, a husband who has recently lost his wife. He develops acute bronchitis, which remains in the chest, and then gets chest pains each time he coughs. The whole heart *chakra* is affected in this case. If he realizes the connection between the loss and bronchitis, healing will occur much faster if he honors the grieving process and treats that as well as the physical ailment.

"You may experience your *chakras* or consciousness centers in meditation, Yoga, Reiki, crystal healing, sound healing, acupuncture, or a variety of different ways. Some people can see the spinning energy in their mind's eye, or they can feel the whirlpool with their hands when they hover their hands over their bodies. Some others feel sensations in their bodies or mental and emotional shifts that correlate with the *chakras*. It is possible to connect with the thoughts and emotions stored in each whirlpool with chakra detection.

"As you begin to feel, sense, or see your *chakras*, their flow may feel underactive or overactive. It may feel deficient and contracted, or spread-out and healthy. A healthy *chakra* system will include *chakras* that are bright in color, balanced in size, and moving at a proper speed.

"Each *chakra* holds the beliefs, emotions, and memories related to specific areas of our life. The lower *chakras* are related to worldly matters such as survival, sex, and power. The top three *chakras* are related to higher consciousness, truth, intuition, and purpose. In the middle, the heart *chakra* bridges the two worlds with empathy, love, and compassion.

"There are many chakras and nadis all over our bodies. There are 114 Chakras and 72,000 nadis. There are seven major chakras, as mentioned above, 21 minor chakras, and 86 micro-chakras in our bodies. Among the 114 chakras, 112 reside in our bodies and two outside it. The minor chakras are present in our hands, legs, tongue, knees, and elbows among other areas. Nadis are a network of subtle energy flows in our bodies. They form the astral and causal bodies. They are the channels and fields of life-energy and consciousness.

"The major seven chakras are as follows.

"Muladhara Chakra

"The *Muladhara,* or Root, Chakra is the *chakra* of stability, security, and our basic needs. It includes the first three vertebrae, the bladder, and the colon. When this *chakra* is open, we feel safe and fearless.

[17]"The Muladhara Chakra symbol consists of a four-petal lotus flower [shaped like] a square and a downward-facing triangle. Each element is said to represent the four aspects of the human mind, uniting to form the birth of the human consciousness. The color is red and represents the Earth. It is located at the base of the spine, between the anus and the genitals. It is characterized by the emotions of survival, stability, ambition, and self-sufficiency.

"When this chakra is out of balance, a person starts feeling unbalanced, ungrounded, with a lack of ambition, lack of purpose, apprehensive, insecure and frustrated. However, when the Muladhara Chakra is balanced, these are replaced by more positive emotions, and you feel balanced, confident, energetic, independent, and strong. The seed mantra (beej mantra) of Muladhara Chakra is 'Lam.'

"Swadhisthana Chakra

"The *Swadhisthana chakra* is our creativity and sexual center. It is located above

[17] *https://www.arhantayoga.org/.*

the pubic bone, below the navel, and is responsible for our creative expression.

"The symbol for the Svadhishthana Chakra or Sacral Chakra is made up of multiple circles, a crescent moon, and six lotus-like-shaped flower petals. The circles and crescent moon represent the recurring nature of life, death, and rebirth, while the six petals portray the six negative aspects of our nature that we need to overcome to open this chakra. The color of this chakra is orange and represents water. It is located in the lower abdomen, about four fingers below the navel. Its attributes include the basic need for sexuality, as well as creativity and self-worth.

"When the Sacral Chakra is imbalanced, a person may feel emotionally explosive and irritable, sense a lack of energy and creativity, feel scheming, or obsessed with sexual thoughts. When balanced, it makes one feel more vibrant, happy, positive, satisfied, compassionate, and intuitive. The seed mantra (beej mantra) of Svadhishthana Chakra is 'Vam.'

"Manipura Chakra

"The *Manipura chakra* means 'lustrous gem' and it's the area from the navel to the breastbone. The third *chakra* is our source of personal power.

"The Manipura, or Solar Plexus, Chakra symbol consists of a downward-pointing triangle within a ten-petalled lotus flower. The ten petals symbolize ten negative character qualities that we have to conquer, while the triangle is the Agni tattva, or fire, of Kundalini energy, which signifies our inner strength. The color associated with this chakra is yellow and represents fire. The Manipura Chakra is located at the solar plexus, between the navel and the bottom of the ribcage. It is characterized by emotions like ego, anger, and aggression.

"An imbalance of the Solar Plexus Chakra can manifest physically as digestive problems, liver problems, or diabetes. On an emotional level, one might struggle with depression, lack of self-esteem, anger, and perfectionism. By balancing this chakra, we feel more energetic, confident, productive, and focused. The seed mantra (beej mantra) of Manipura Chakra is 'Ram.'

"Anahata Chakra

"Located at the heart center, the fourth *chakra*, Anahata, is in the middle of the seven and unites the lower *chakras* of matter and the upper *chakras* of spirit.

The fourth is also spiritual but serves as a bridge between our body, mind, emotions, and spirit. The heart *chakra* is our source of love and connection. When we work through our physical *chakras*, or the first three, we can open the spiritual *chakras* more fully.

"In the Anahata, or the Heart, Chakra symbol, two triangles intersect to form a yantra, which represents the balance of yin and yang, or upward and downward forces. Outside, there is a lotus flower with twelve petals symbolizing the twelve divine qualities associated with the heart. The color associated with this chakra is green and represents the element of air. As the name implies, the Anahata Chakra is located in the heart region. This chakra is the seat of balance, and it is characterized by emotions of love, attachment, compassion, trust, and passion.

"When the heart chakra is imbalanced, a person may deal with emotional issues like anger, lack of trust, anxiety, jealousy, fear, and moodiness.

"By making this energy center harmonious, a person begins to feel more compassionate, caring, optimistic, friendly, and motivated. The seed mantra (beej mantra) of Anahata Chakra is 'Yam.'

"Vishuddha Chakra

"The *Vishuddha chakra* is the fifth *chakra*, located in the area of the throat. This is our source of verbal expression and the ability to speak our highest truth. The fifth *chakra* includes the neck, thyroid and parathyroid glands, jaw, mouth, and tongue.

"The symbol of the Throat Chakra consists of a sixteen-petalled lotus flower surrounding an inverted triangle, which holds a circle within. This represents spiritual growth and the purification of the body, mind, and spirit. The color associated with this chakra is blue and represents the element of space. The Visuddha Chakra is located at the base of the throat, coinciding with the thyroid gland. It is associated with inspiration, healthy expression, faith, and good communication.

"A blockage in the throat chakra may be experienced as nervousness, quietness, a feeling of weakness, or the inability to express our thoughts. When this chakra is balanced, it enables creativity, positive self-expression, constructive communication, and a sense of satisfaction.

"The seed mantra (beej mantra) of Vishuddha Chakra is 'Ham.'

"Ajna Chakra

"The *Ajna chakra* is located in between the eyebrows. It is also referred to as the third eye chakra. *Ajna* is our center of intuition. We all have a sense of intuition but we may ignore it many times to our peril. An effort on opening the sixth *chakra* will help you improve this ability.

The Third Eye Chakra symbol consists of an inverted triangle resting in a circle between two lotus petals. The two petals and downward-facing pyramid both signify wisdom, emphasizing the Third Eye Chakra's role in our journey to spiritual awareness. Its color is Indigo and does not represent any element. The Ajna Chakra (pronounced as 'Agya Chakra') is located between the eyebrows. Also known as the Third Eye Chakra, it is often used as a main point during asana practice to develop more concentration and awareness. It is said that meditating upon this chakra destroys the karma of past lives and brings liberation and intuitive wisdom. Its attributes are intelligence, intuition, insight, and self-knowledge.

"When imbalanced, it may make you feel non-emphatic and afraid of success, or on the contrary, it can make you more egoistic. An imbalance can manifest as physical problems like headaches, blurry vision, and eye strain.

"When this chakra is active and balanced, a person feels more vibrant and confident, both spiritually and emotionally. In the absence of the fear of death, one becomes his own master and remains free of all attachment to material things. The seed mantra (beej mantra) of Ajna Chakra is 'Om.'

"Sahasrara Chakra

"The *Sahasrara chakra,* or the "thousand-petal lotus," *chakra* is located at the crown of the head. This is the *chakra* of enlightenment and spiritual connection to our higher selves, others, and ultimately, to the Lord. It is located at the crown of the head.

"The Crown Chakra symbol is depicted as a ring of a thousand lotus petals surrounding an inverted triangle. This symbolizes the rising of divine energy into the Crown Chakra, bringing spiritual liberation and enlightenment. The color associated with this chakra is violet white and does not represent any elements. The Sahastrara, or Crown, Chakra is located at the crown of the head. The seventh chakra is the center of spirituality, enlightenment, and vibrant thought and energy. It allows for the inward flow of wisdom and brings the reward of cosmic consciousness.

"When it gets imbalanced, one might suffer from a constant sense of frustration, melancholy and destructive feelings. A balanced Crown Chakra promotes spiritual realization, internal peace and a clear viewpoint on the world. The seed mantra (beej mantra) of Sahastrara Chakra is 'Aum.'

"Awareness to which of your *chakras* are out of balance is key to aligning them. Our bodies are in constant flux between balance and imbalance. Unless you experience an apparent problem in one area of the body, imbalances can be difficult to detect. However, it's good to bring pure awareness to your body/mind and start understanding its signals and clues so that you can align your *chakras*. For example, frequent constipation can indicate a blockage in the first *chakra*. A recurring sore throat leaves clues to a blocked fifth *chakra*. Frequent headaches around the area of the forehead may mean your sixth *chakra* is blocked.

"When healing the *chakras*, it's better to commence with the root *chakra*, and search ideas related to protection, nourishment, belonging, finances, and family. From there, you may move up the spine to the sacral *chakra* and so forth. The health of the lower *chakras* is crucial to the health of the upper *chakras*. Without a sense of grounding, stability, and safety, it may feel jolting to open up the third eye or crown *chakras* that are related to intuition, divine linking, and higher wisdom."

I stopped and took a long sip of the refilled orange juice and also took a bite of a cookie. We sat in silence for a while, after which Madhu asked, "Shomikda, there are so many wonders of our own bodies and existence, isn't it? Our education system teaches nothing about that."

I said, "That is unfortunately true in the modern world. We have learnt to explore the physical body but have neglected the inner coverings of our existence. That was taught in ancient India in the Gurukuls, but now everything seems to be going south about understanding one's entire existence. However, in recent times, some inkling of a revival seems to be visible. Let us see what unfolds in this sequence of history of civilization."

"Let me tell you about Sree Padmanabha Temple, where I visited in South India," Madhu said after a little more remaining in silence for some more time.

He continued, [18]"The origin of the Temple of Sree Padmanabhaswamy is

---

[18] *https://spst.in/temple.*

lost in antiquity. It is not possible to determine with any exactitude, from any reliable historical documents or other sources as to when and by whom the original idol of Sree Padmanabhaswamy was consecrated. The Temple has references in Epics and Puranas. Srimad Bhagavatha says that Balarama visited this Temple, bathed in Padmatheertham and made several offerings. Nammalwar, 9th Century poet and one among the twelve Vaishnavite saints of the Alvar tradition, has composed ten hymns in praise of Lord Padmanabha. Some well-known scholars, writers and historians, like the late Dr. L.A.Ravi Varma of Travancore, have expressed the view that this Temple was established on the first day of Kali Yuga (which was over five thousand years ago). The legends of the Temple are handed down through the centuries. One such legend that finds a place in the old palm leaf records of the Temple, as also in the famous grantha entitled 'Ananthasayana Mahatmya,' mentions that it was consecrated by a Tulu Brahmin hermit named Divakara Muni. On the 950th year of Kali Yuga a reinstallation of the idol was done. In the 960th Kali year King Kotha Marthandan built the Abhisravana Mandapam.

"The story as narrated in the Ananthasayana Mahatmya goes as follows:

"Divakara Muni was a great Vishnu devotee. While at 'Aanarthadesa,' he performed deep tapas. One day Maha Vishnu appeared before the sage as a lovely child. The charming child attracted the attention of the sage. He requested the God-child to stay with him. The child made his stay conditional. Accordingly, the Sanyasi should treat him with respect. On failing to do so, he would vanish at once. This was accepted and the child stayed with him. The hermit gave him great care and tolerated the childish pranks. One day, when the sanyasi was in deep meditation at his prayers, the chills took the 'salagram,' which the sanyasi was using for worship, and put it into his mouth and made such a nuisance of himself that Divakara Mini was greatly angered and could tolerate it no further. He thereupon chastised the child. In accordance with the earlier agreement, immediately the child ran away and disappeared from the spot. While going he said, 'If you wish to see me again, you will find me again in Ananthankaadu.' It was only then that Divakara Muni realized who his erstwhile child guest had been. The hermit was stricken with inconsolable grief and for many days followed what he believed was the route taken by the child foregoing food, rest and sleep in the process.

"Finally, he reached a wooded area near the seacoast, caught a glimpse of the child disappearing into a huge 'Ilappa' tree. Immediately the tree fell into the ground and it assumed the form of Sree Maha Vishnu. The divine form had its head at 'Thiruvallam' (a place about three miles from East Fort, where the Temple of Sree Padmanabha Swamy is located) and its feet at 'Trippapur' (five miles away toward the north). Overawed by the majesty and the size of the divine form, which manifested before him, the Sanyasi prayed to the Lord to condense Himself in size so that he could behold Him. There upon the image of the Lord shrank to a size, three times the length of the Sanyasi's Yoga Dand. His prayers had been granted. He immediately offered a raw mango in a coconut shell (still this offering continues). The Lord ordained that poojas to Him should be conducted by Tulu Brahmins. To this day half the number of poojaris (priests) in this Temple represent Tulu region. Another generally accepted version about the origin of the Temple relates it to the famous Namboothiri sanyasi Vilvamangalathu Swamiyar, whose name is linked with the histories of several temples in Southern India. This Swamiyar was also a Vishnu devotee. The legend is almost identical to that of Divakara Muni referred above. It is said that when Sree Maha Vishnu presented himself in the Ananthasayana rupa (in the form of reclining on Anantha) before the sage at Ananthankaadu, the latter had nothing worthwhile to offer Him. From a mango tree standing nearby he plucked a few unripe mangoes and placed them in a coconut shell lying there and in all humility offered it as 'nivedyam' to the Lord. Even today salted mango forms a major offering. The original coconut shell has been encased in gold. It has also been the practice in the Temple for the past several centuries that the morning 'pushpanjali' is to be performed by a Namboothiri Brahmin sanyasi (designated Pushpanjali Swamiyar) specially commissioned for this purpose.

"These traditional customs coupled with the fact that the Pushpanjali Swamiyar holds a position of importance in the 'Ettara Yogam' (a committee which, at one time in the distant past, was the governing body of the Temple but has, over the years, become a ceremonial and advisory panel) lend substance and some measures of credence to the theory that this Temple was founded by Vilvamangalathu Swamiyar. On the other hand, the legend of the Divakara Muni can be substantiated by the presence of a large number of Tulu Brahmins. Besides being represented in the 'Yogam,' the Namboothiri Brahmins also have a position of eminence in the rituals and ceremonies of the Temple. The Tantric (high priests) have always been from the Tharananalloor family belonging to this community. It is also believed that the small Sree Krishna Swamy Temple, located near the Western Swamiyar Madham (residence of one of the two Pushpanjali Swamiyars of the Temple), has been built over the Samadhi of Vilvamangalathu Swamiyar. Some historians and researchers hold the view that the Thiruvambadi shrine of Sree Krishna Swamy is older than the shrine of Sree Padmanabhaswamy. According to legend the Sree Narasimhaswamy and Sree Sastha shrines were established after the installation of the idol of Lord Sree Padmanabhaswamy. There is mention in the 'Bhagavatha Purana' (canto 10, chapter 79) that Sree Balarama visited 'Syanandoorapuram' or 'Ananthasayam' (Thiruvananthapuram) in the course of His pilgrimage. Similarly, in the 'Brahmanda Purana' also there is a reference to 'Syanandoorapura.' These references show that this Temple is of great antiquity and has been held in veneration over the centuries as an important seat of Sree Maha Vishnu. The compositions of Nammalvar, the great Vaishnavite saint, in praise of Sree Maha Vishnu of this city prove beyond doubt that this Temple existed in the ninth century of this era. In the year 1050A.D. (225M.E.), the Temple was reconstructed and the management reorganized by the then ruler.

"The next important recorded events relate to the period between 1335 A.D. and 1384 A.D., when Venad was ruled by a powerful and wise king named Veera Marthanda Varma. He gradually established his authority completely over the management and administration of the Temple. There are records to indicate that in the year 1375 A.D. the Alpasi Utsavam (ten-day festival held in October-November) was conducted in the Temple. In 1728 A.D. propitiatory ceremonies, connected with the serious fire of 1686, were conducted.

"It was in the year 1729 that the great ruler Marthanda Varma became the king of Travancore. He took the steps to renovate the Temple. In 1730 the idol was again moved to 'Balalaya' prior to the renovation and reconstruction of the sanctum sanctorum. It took two years for completion. The old wooden idol was replaced by the one that we see today. Made of highly complex amalgam known as Katusarkarayogam, it contains 12,008 Salagrams within it. Most of what is seen today within the walls of the temple was constructed. It is recorded that four thousand sculptors, six thousand laborers and one hundred elephants worked for a period of six months to finish the construction of the sreebalippura (the oblong corridor). This magnificent rectangular corridor built of solid stones protects the Deities during seeveli on rainy days. The gopuram, for which the foundation had been laid in 1566, was built during this period. Similarly, the flagstaff in front of the main shrine was also erected at this time. Teak wood of the required size was brought from the forest for this purpose and transported to the Temple in such a way that no part of the wood touched the ground. The pole was then covered completely with gold sheets. The renovation of the Temple tank, the Padmatheertham, including the flight steps and its completion in the form we see it today, was also undertaken during this great ruler's time.

"The temple is the wealthiest place of worship in the world, having treasure collected over millennia in six hitherto known vaults (nilavaras), labelled as A to F. In April 2014, reportedly two more subterranean vaults, which had been named G and H, were found. While vault B has been unopened over centuries, vaults A, C, D, E, and F were opened along with some of their antechambers. Among the reported findings are a three-and-a-half foot-tall solid pure golden idol of Mahavishnu, studded with hundreds of diamonds and rubies and other precious stones. Also found were an eighteen-foot-long pure gold chain, a gold sheaf weighing 500 kilograms (1,100 pounds), a 36-kilogram (79-pound) golden veil, 1200 'Sarappalli' gold coin-chains that are encrusted with precious stones, and several sacks filled with golden artefacts, necklaces, diadems, diamonds, rubies, sapphires, emeralds, gemstones, and objects made of other precious metals. Ceremonial attire for adorning the deity in the form of sixteen-part gold anki weighing almost 30 kilograms (66 pounds), gold 'coconut shells' studded with rubies and emeralds, and several 18th Century Napoleonic-era coins were found amongst many other objects. In early 2012, an expert committee had been appointed to investigate these objects, which include lakhs of golden coins of the Roman Empire that were found in Kottayam, in Kannur District. According to Vinod Rai, the former Comptroller-and-Auditor-General (CAG) of India, who had audited some of the Temple records from 1990, in August 2014, in the already opened vault A, there is an 800-kilogram (1,800-pound) hoard of gold coins dating to around 200 B.C.E., each coin priced at over US$340,000. Also found was a pure golden throne, studded with hundreds of diamonds and other precious stones, meant for the eighteen-foot-long deity. As per one of the men, who was among those that went inside this vault, a several of the largest diamonds were as large as a full-grown man's thumb. According to varying reports, at least three, if not more, solid gold crowns have been found, studded with diamonds and other precious stones. Some other media reports also mention hundreds of pure gold chairs, thousands of gold pots and jars, among the articles recovered from vault A and its antechambers. The total value will be estimated to be over an estimated trillion U.S. dollars."

Madhu gave this compelling account of the richest place of worship, Sree Padmanabha Temple, which proves that India was the richest country in the world having over 33% of the share of GDP till about 10th Century A.D.

We sat and allowed the information to sink in, filling us with a sense of pride to ruminate on our glorious ancient past.

The day was going into the early afternoon and I decided to call it a day and go back home. My wife was waiting for me after having cooked our lunch in the morning. So, I bid Madhu goodbye until next time.

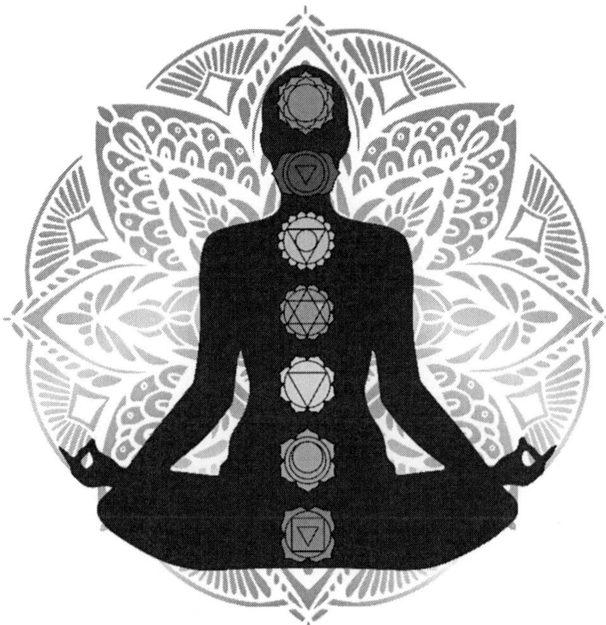

Seven chakras on meditating yogi man silhouette. Credit: littlepaw

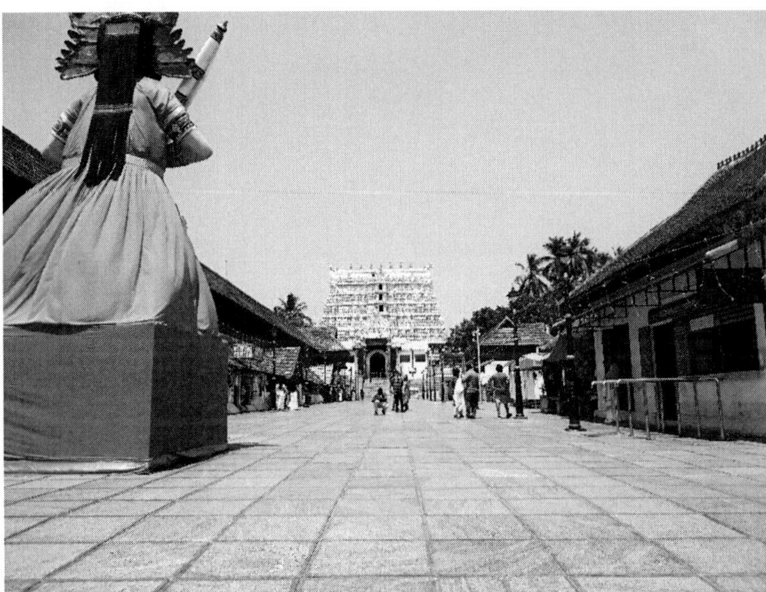

Sri Padmanabhaswamy Temple of Trivandrum or Thiruvananthapuram in day light, people going to worship or pray. Credit: sisyphuszirix

Chapter 4

The Mystery of Consciousness

"Shomikda, what is consciousness?"

Madhu sipped on a cup of tea in our house while discussing this most intriguing question on our existence.

I thought for a while before saying, "There are various theories of consciousness in the scientific world, none of which are conclusive. According to an article entitled [19]'What is Consciousness,' which had a theory called IIT, or Integrated Information Theory, states, 'consciousness is intrinsic causal power associated with complex mechanisms such as the human brain.'

"IIT theory also derives from the complexity of the underlying interconnected structure, a single nonnegative number Φ (pronounced "*fy*") that quantifies this consciousness. If Φ is zero, the system does not feel like anything to be itself. Conversely, the bigger this number, the more intrinsic causal power the system possesses and the more conscious it is. The brain, which has enormous and highly specific connectivity, possesses very high Φ, which implies a high level of consciousness. IIT explains a number of observations, such as why the cerebellum does not contribute to consciousness and why the zap-and-zip meter works. (The quantity the meter measures is a very crude approximation of Φ.)

[20]"I also read an interesting article on consciousness. When I am writing, my hand and fingers function very consciously. The same hand and fingers

[19] "What Is Consciousness?" in *Scientific American* 318, 6, 60-64 (June 2018). Doi: 10.1038/scientificamerican0618-60.

[20] Writings of Dr. Harish Mehta.

will not be as conscious when I will be deep in sleep in the middle of the night that somebody may even lift my hand and shift it to another place without my being aware of it. In other words, the hand and fingers exhibit consciousness during the day but not in deep sleep, though their gross chemistry continues to take place, such as the blood circulation, etc. This leads us to think that the consciousness that the hand and fingers exhibited was not their own property. It was borrowed by them from another entity. That is to say, there is another entity that has the inherent property of consciousness. Let us call it C for the time being. C is the source of consciousness and it lends its consciousness to the hand and fingers during the daytime. This concept of another entity C different from the body, though living in the body, is further strengthened by the fact that a person lives consciously even after a significant number of body organs are missing. For example, a person will remain alive and conscious without any change whatsoever to his consciousness even if his hands and feet are chopped off. From the body perspective, this is a significant change but the person remains the same—the person as a conscious being hasn't changed by an iota, though the body has undergone major changes. The same applies to the people who were severely burnt and are still alive; their body has undergone a massive change but the person remains the same. This proves that we are something beyond the body and that something has the property of consciousness.

"The above indicates that the body inhabits another entity that has consciousness as its intrinsic and inherent property, what we have temporarily called as C. Before we give it a more acceptable name, we must explore its nature to some extent. The first thing that comes in mind is that it must be different from the body in certain respects. Indeed, the moment a person dies, the body is more or less the same in the very next moment but consciousness has disappeared forever. So, C must be a non-material thing, markedly different from the body frame, and also it must be so because consciousness is absent in the myriads of material things that we see around us. Therefore, we can say that besides material things in the world, there must be a non-material thing that has consciousness. Thus, C is a non-material thing. We can call it our true spirit, our soul. As long as it resides in the body, I have life. Its union with the body was my birth and its separation from the body will be death.

"Some other theories propound that the universe is indeed conscious.

[21]"The mathematics is such that if something is conscious according to the theory, then the components that make up that system can't have conscious experiences on their own. Only the whole has conscious experience, not the parts. Applied to your brain, it means that some of your cortex might be conscious but the particles that make up the cortex are not themselves conscious.

"My take on this subject is that consciousness is the non-physical energy that makes us aware. It is an awareness energy that is non-physical in nature that pervades the whole creation. The entire creation comes out of that and dissolves into that at the end of the cycle.

"'If there is an isolated pair of particles floating around somewhere in space, they will have some rudimentary form of consciousness if they interact in the correct way,' said a scientist.

"According to Integrated Information Theory, the universe is indeed full of consciousness. But does it have implications for the physical part of the universe? The math of the theory says it does not. A physical system will operate independently, whether it has a conscious experience or not.

"From the above discussions, it is apparent that the Western scientists still do not have a comprehensive grasp on the nature of consciousness. Our Indian rishis had understood the nature of consciousness many thousands of years ago and were initially orally passed down and subsequently written down for future generations to learn and understand the nature of Creation. Vedantha explains it lucidly.

"The Vedantha philosophy has considered mind as the subtle form of matter wherein the body and its components are considered the grossest forms. Consciousness, on the other hand, is considered finer than 'mind matter' and is considered all pervasive, omnipresent and omniscient. The ancient seers (the rishis) claimed that such truths are revealed only by intuitive research by diving deep into the self in the process of absorption (Samadhi)."

I took a sip on the coffee cup to fill myself with reinvigorating liquid, commonly referred in New York at least as "Joe." "Have a cup of Joe" is what people tell each other.

My wife had also placed a plate of hot samosas for us to enjoy while having a serious discussion on this complicated topic.

---

[21] Can our brains help prove the universe is conscious? By David Crookes, *All About Space* magazine, published February 23, 2022.

After a couple of bites of the samosa, I continued. "I believe that the entire creation is conscious. But every particle has its own level of consciousness. Let me describe to you the flowering of consciousness.

"The Vedic Scriptures divide consciousness into five categories, namely covered, shrunken, budding, blooming and fully bloomed.

"Trees, plants, for example, are almost inert. They fall into the 'covered consciousness' category. They seem to show no sign of consciousness, but when we observe them carefully, we see they have a limited consciousness. Even the so-called non-living things have a limited consciousness. Indian scientist Jagadish Chandra Bose, who discovered that plants have life and also arguably, the radio, experimented on some tin cans, among others, and showed that they reacted to being beaten by a hammer through a microscope.

"Other living entities, such as worms, insects, and other animals, are in 'shrunken consciousness.' They are not as covered as the plants, but their consciousness is not fully developed either.

"Human beings have 'budding consciousness.' A bud appears shrunken, but it has the potential to bloom into a flower. Human consciousness has similar potential; it appears shrunken like the animals, but humans have the innate ability to develop their consciousness to an almost unlimited extent, up to the point of knowing the Absolute Truth, the Supreme Personality of Godhead or Paramatma, Parabrahma.

"Other species do not have this special ability. That is why the Vedic scriptures consider the human form of life as the most elevated. Indeed, all scriptures consider human life especially sacred.

"When a human being begins to inquire sincerely about the Absolute Truth, his budlike spiritual consciousness begins to expand or evolve. That is the 'blooming consciousness.' When as a result of his inquiry he practices regulated spiritual discipline, he evolves further and further. Finally, he attains the 'fully bloomed' state of consciousness.

"God realization is possible because a living being is spirit soul, not the material body. The soul is not a product of material nature, it comes from our spiritual nature. When the soul falls into the lower levels of consciousness, it becomes covered by matter—first by a subtle, or ethereal, material body made of mind, intelligence and false ego, then by a gross material body made of earth, water, fire, air and ether.

"The bodies we perceive with our material vision are gross material bodies. Within the gross body is the subtle body, which we cannot see with our eyes but can perceive by our intelligence.

"Finer than this subtle material body of mind, intelligence and false ego is the nonmaterial soul, which animates the body. The soul is the source of consciousness, the source of life in the body. The soul is the 'I.'

"As long as the soul is in the body, the body appears alive, consciousness flows through the body, and the covered soul misidentifies the body as the self.

"An embodied soul transmigrates from one body to another as a result of his previous karma. His every action leaves an imprint on the mind, or the subtle body, and accordingly the subtle body takes its shape.

"For example, if one acts like an angel, his subtle body becomes like that of an angel. If one acts like a pig, his subtle body becomes like that of a pig. When the soul leaves the gross body at death, the subtle body carries the soul to an appropriate womb determined by the shape of the subtle body. In this way the soul transmigrates from one body to another according to the state of consciousness it has developed.

"The Vedic scriptures describe that one gets a human body after transmigrating through eight million lower species. Gradually each fallen soul evolves through the various stages of consciousness—covered, shrunken, and budding. At the budding stage the embodied soul has the chance to develop fully his spiritual consciousness by awakening his relationship with God, the supremely conscious being. If he neglects that opportunity, he may again undergo transmigration through the covered, shrunken and budding stages.

"The subhuman species are engrossed in bodily consciousness. Often human beings are also, but human beings can raise themselves to higher levels. That is the main difference between man and the animals. If a man, in spite of his higher faculties, simply pursues the animal propensities of eating, sleeping, mating, and defending, he grossly misuses a wonderful gift. He misses a rare opportunity.

"A human being, because of his elevated intelligence, has the freedom to choose, either to evolve spiritually and get out of material consciousness altogether or to go down to lower consciousness again.

"Less intelligent persons often consider sensual enjoyment the goal of life and squander their lives struggling for objects pleasing to their senses. Their absorption in material ambitions at the expense of spiritual upliftment makes lower consciousness their choice by default.

"Intelligent persons realize the futility of such endeavors for bodily pleasures. They realize that everything in the material realm is temporary. By finer intelligence they understand that all attempts to enjoy end in bondage and misery. That's why throughout history our greatest thinkers were averse to material enjoyments without limitations.

"A truly intelligent person, therefore, tries to find the standard of real enjoyment. If such a person is serious and has good fortune he comes in touch with a genuine God-realized spiritual master from whom he learns what real enjoyment is. With the spiritual master's guidance, he gets the opportunity to reestablish his long-lost relationship with God.

"This awakening of the soul's dormant love of God is an absolute necessity because the soul, as a spark-like part of God, is never fully satisfied unless united with Him. This is the central message of the Vedic texts.

"If one wants to taste real pleasure, he must develop spiritual consciousness, which culminates in love of God. That is the topmost state of consciousness, consciousness in full bloom. It is the ultimate evolution of man, not only for today, but for all time."

Madhu, who was listening intently to my talk, gave out a sigh of resignation and said sadly, "Will I ever get to the high planes of consciousness? It seems so far."

"If we make small steps every moment, then one day we will reach our destination. Practice every day, if not every moment. You will see the transformation in you," I said reassuringly.

After eating our share of samosas and tea/coffee, Madhu started on cue.

"Shomikda, another beautiful temple that I visited was the [22]Ranganathaswamy Temple in Srirangam in Tamil Nadu. It is the largest temple complex in India. This temple is one of the rare self-manifested temples of Lord Vishnu. It follows and worships the Thenkalai tradition of Sri Vaishnavism.

"The temple is also known as the world's largest functioning Hindu temple complex. It is also one of the most important of the 108 Divya Desams, or Vishnu temples. It is also the resting place of Lord Vishnu and has over eighty shrines of Goddesses Laxmi and Saraswati, among other deities across the complex.

"The temple complex is built on 156 acres of land. It has seven enclosures. These enclosures are formed by tall, thick rampart walls running around the sanctum. There are twenty-one towers, or gopurams, in all enclosures decreas-

[22] *Incredibleindia.com.*

ing in height inwards. The temple town lies on an islet formed by the rivers Kaveri and Kollidam.

"The gopuram on the southern side of the temple, called the Rajagopuram, is 239.5 feet tall and, as of 2016, is the tallest in Asia. The construction of the Rajagopuram began during the reign of Achyuta Deva Raya of the Vijayanagara Empire. However, construction was halted after his death and the structure of the Rajagopuram remained incomplete for over four hundred years. The completion of the Rajagopuram was undertaken and completed successfully by Sri Vedanta Desika Yatheendra Mahadesikan, the 44th jeeyar of Sri Ahobila Matha. The construction spanned eight years before it was consecrated on 25 March 1987.

"In historic times, just after the construction of this temple, the city of Srirangam lived completely within the walls of this temple and is often described as a religious utopia.

"The Ranganathaswamy temple is one of the three temples of the God Ranganatha (Antya Ranga) that are situated in the natural islands formed in the Kaveri River. They are:

Adi Ranga: the Sri Ranganathaswamy Temple at Srirangapatna, Srirangapatna taluk, Mandya district, Karnataka, India

Madhya Ranga: the Sri Ranganathaswamy Temple at Shivanasamudra, Kollegala taluk, Chamarajanagara district, Karnataka, India

Antya Ranga: the Sri Ranganathaswamy Temple at Srirangam, Srirangam taluk, Tiruchirappalli district, Tamil Nadu, India.

"There is a gopuram fully made of gold, which is protected by an electrical fence. Clothes such as silk sarees, dhoti and towels, which are used for religious purposes, are auctioned here.

"Saint Ramanuja, the 11th century saint, one of the most celebrated theologians of Hinduism, made his monastic home by the temple at Srirangam. Here he wrote his famous commentaries on the *Brahma Sutra*, which expressed a qualified non-dualism of the Vedanta, his Vishishtadvaita. Ramanuja's body is said to come out of the Earth after he was buried and was preserved at this temple. Although Ramanuja hailed from Sriperumbudur and a pivotal point in his lifetime, receiving the Ashtakshara mantram, happened in Thirukoshtiyur, he made Srirangam his home after the demise of his Acharya in spirit, Alavanthar, or Yamunacharya."

"Madhu, you are so fortunate to visit such iconic monuments and temples of our ancient past that exemplify our advanced civilization and prosperity in the ancient past. Ancient temples were built differently. They used the energy outlets of the earth to construct temples with consecrated deities to enable regular people to experience the tremendous energy that envelops the area. Temple construction is science and art. It is used to enhance the spiritual energy of people and was used in ancient temples especially. People should always visit ancient temples and drink the energy," I said with conviction.

Another day of exciting conversation came to an end. Madhu tread toward the door with a reassuring smile that he would be back.

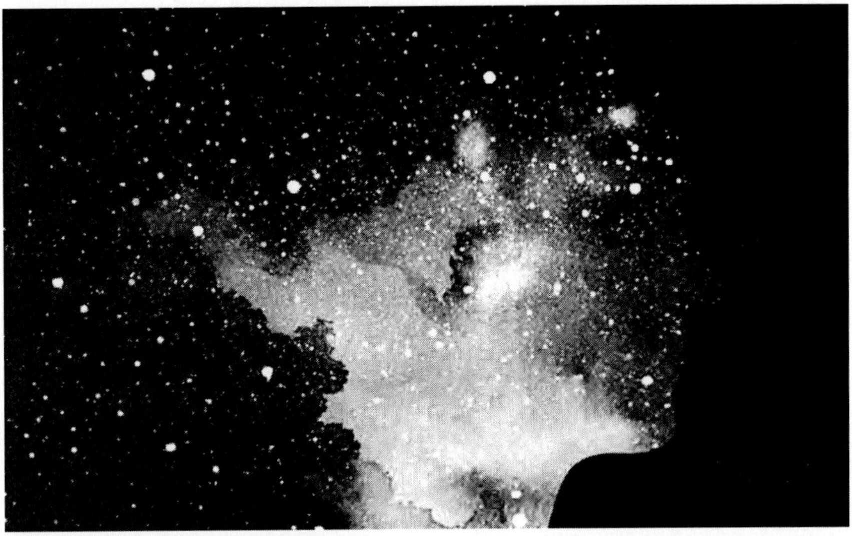

Vector illustration of human head on starry space background. Artificial intelligence or cosmic consciousness. Credit: WhataWin

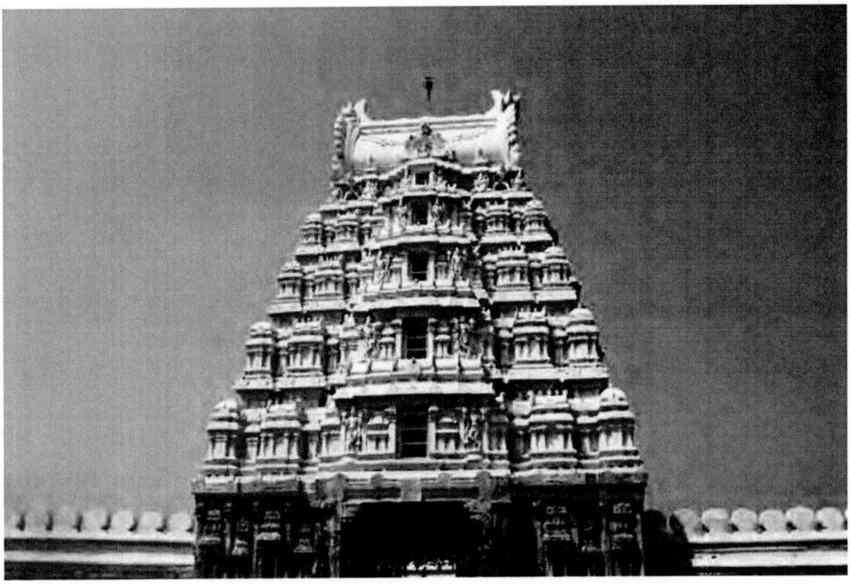

Gopuram of the Ranganathaswamy Temple, located inside the fort is believed to have been built by Ramanuja, Srirangapatna, Karnataka. Credit: vbel71

Chapter 5
Human Potential

Madhu came to our house again the following weekend. We sat with airs of resignation and relaxation. Until Madhu said, "Shomikda, please tell me about human potential that you talk about at times."

That was the spark that I needed to start my incessant talk. I smiled and said, "The magnificent creation of the Lord that expands beyond the comprehension of humanity has been the topic of much speculation and debate for millennia. Peering into the dark infinity, people have tried to fathom the mysteries behind this vast existence. But with the stark limitations of physical matter and energies associated with it, it is an impossible task to unravel most of the mysteries that surround us all around.

"Against all theories that modern scientists have developed about human evolution and the passage of history, it is interesting to know that human existence was much more developed in certain ways in ages far beyond the knowledge of modern man. I do not intend to undertake a lecture on the history of evolution, but there are some astounding pages of wisdom that are encrypted in the Vedic scriptures that profess the same.

"In recent times, modern special photography has given one of the many material proofs of what our Vedic sages of wisdom had been telling for millennia far before the existence of Mesopotamia, Babylon, Egypt or any other civilization. Modern special photography has shown that every living creature on this planet has an aura around himself or herself that gives the characteristics, physical, mental, emotional and spiritual state of that person. A personal trait can be determined from that and even diseases could be identified and cured.

"According to our scriptures, the spirit is enclosed in a body-mind complex comprising of five sheaths called the Pancha Kosas. They are Annamaya Kosa, the food or the material body sheath; Pranamaya Kosa, the vital-air sheath; Manomaya Kosa, the mental sheath; Vignanamaya Kosa, the intellectual sheath; and Anandamaya Kosa, the bliss sheath.

"The soul, spirit or atma is distinct from this sheath and is the spark of the Absolute or God.

"Annamaya Kosa, or Sthula Sarira, is the gross body made up of the five elements—earth, fire, water, air, and space. Pranamayam, Manomaya and Vignanamaya Kosas constitute the subtle body or the Sukshma Sarira, and Anandamaya Kosa is the causal body or the Karana Sarira embedding vasanas (inclinations and tendencies), which cause human birth.

"Our physical body is made up of bones, muscles, blood vessels and other constituents but is coordinated, run and maintained by the brain in association with the spinal cord, which are jointly termed as the central nervous system of our physical body. It is that part that gives life to the otherwise lump of flesh and bones.

"Unlimited Human Potential

"Our sages have said for thousands of years about the infinite potentiality of every human being. In Indian spiritual culture or Hinduism, we are seekers, not believers. We seek out the truth through austerities. Our foundation is based on Cosmic Laws or Dharma. So, we arouse this potential energy that could raise us from the state of a rational animal to the divine state, which is the original and perfect state of existence for all creatures. The door to that state lies at the base of our spinal cord and is called Kula Kundalini, or Kundalini, an infinite potential energy that is represented as three-and-a-half coils of a sleeping serpent. A small part of Kundalini is the life force that we have, but the majority is an immense energy potential at the base of the spine.

"Kundalini in the form of a 'coiled snake' is a form of divine feminine energy (or Shakti) located at the base of the spine, below the Muladhara chakra. In Haiva Tantra, where it is believed to be a force or power associated with the divine feminine or the formless aspect of the goddess. This energy in the body, when cultivated and awakened through spiritual practice, is believed to lead to 'Moksha,' or spiritual liberation. Kuṇḍalinī is associated with Parvati or Adi Parashakti, the Supreme Being in Shaktism, and with the goddesses Bhairavi and Kubjika. The term, along with practices associated with it, was adopted into Hatha Yoga in the later years. It has since then been adopted into other forms of Hinduism as well as modern spirituality and New Age thought. "Kuṇḍalini awakenings concentrate on awakening Kuṇḍalini through meditation, pranayama breathing mainly, and also the practice of asana and chanting of mantras. Kundalini Yoga is influenced by Shaktism and Tantra schools of Hinduism. It derives its name from its focus upon the awakening of Kundalini energy through regular practice of Mantra, Tantra, Yantra, Asanas and Meditation.

"When the Kundalini is aroused, there are two ways of its journey. One is the material movement, which expresses itself in sex. It is wastage of the prized energy. The rishis controlled the physical waste of energy and helped it to rise up the Sushumna, which is a very thin passage or ethereal cord running through the spine of the subtle body. This is similar to the spinal cord of the physical body. This vast energy produces frequencies that cannot be produced by our physical bodies or by external energy sources. The subtle nerves get energized and the person can uplift his consciousness from the physical level to a much more elevated level. It is a long and arduous journey filled with pitfalls and distractions. The ultimate state of attainment would take many, many lives and is a journey through one body to the next and next.

"This journey to the spiritual world is considered by the Vedic literature to be a natural journey back home. It also states that only 10 percent of the entire creation is the material world, while 90 percent constitutes the spiritual world. So, we see how small this infinite material world is in comparison to the actual creation.

"To arouse the Kundalini, we need to follow certain procedures and practices that have been time tested for thousands of years. We also need to follow certain principles like continence, purity, and cleanliness among others. Most importantly, we have to develop devotion and love of God to attain the highest stages of existence as without that, a sadhaka or person doing austerities, can easily fall prey to the ego and other pitfalls during the journey.

"The Process of Self-Realization[23]

"When a paper is put under a magnifying glass and the sun's rays are focused on the paper, the paper starts to burn. Similarly, if we practice concentrating

[23] Lectures from famous author and spiritual saint Sarkarkaku, or "Nigurananda," or Prof. Satchidananda Sarkar, who used to come to our house regularly for years, explaining all that he saw in meditation.

deeply in between our eyebrows, then the Kundalini gets aroused slowly. Thereafter, it starts to go up the Sushumna cord like mercury rising up the pressure monitor. To attain concentration, sit comfortably and close your eyes and stare in front of your eyes like you do at the movie theaters. If you remember, at the movie theaters, once you stare at the screen in front, you lose awareness of your surroundings. Slowly, concentration will develop and you will lose awareness of the surroundings.

"This energy allows us to generate those vibrations that are impossible to attain by normal physical means. The Sushumna cord has six centers or plexuses through which the energy must flow to reach the crown plexus on the top of the brain.

"Kundalini Yoga is a method that has been nurtured by mixing the micro, or the earth, and the macro, or the heavenly cosmos. This is micro-macro parallelism. The individual being and the Universal Being are one.

"The first stage, or the Muladhara Chakra, situated at the base of the spine, is the first plexus to be passed. The person experiences tremors and sees colors, including red. In most circumstances, he should be able to see a spark of light, which is the 'Light of God,' or the 'Bindu of Omkar.' However, many would just see darkness initially. But the persistence with meditation is a must and slowly he will see one or multiple lights. He has to focus on one light and that will lead him on to the higher realms.

"Fixing his concentration on the light, he would move on to the next plexus Swadhistana Chakra, which lies at the level of the genital organs two inches above the Muladhara Chakra. He would see colors where red turns to green and various other things but all in a haze. On further concentration and practice, he would rise up to Manipura Chakra, or the navel wheel. Here, he would see a haze of white light and various other lights and holy symbols.

"After much penance, the sadhaka is able to rise from the Manipura Chakra to the Anahata Chakra, or the heart wheel. It is the transition from the bondage of the material world to a rise toward the spiritual world. The person would be sucked into a giant black hole, which can be terrifying, but with devotion and faith in the Lord and following the ever-increasing spark of light, he would reach, with a start, a serene sky of blue where he would float like a bird in the sky (Brihangam Yoga). Visions would become clearer to him and he would start getting a taste of the divinity that is innate in him.

"Moving further on, the Kundalini rises to the Vishuddi Chakra, or the laryngeal wheel, where the sadhaka experiences the bliss of divinity in abundance. Blue color becomes dark blue and visions of various states of evolution, gods and goddesses, various expansions of the Supreme Lord who runs the universes in their subtle forms, visions of the past, present and future that is imprinted on the 'photo negative' of the Lord's subtle expanse, mysteries of creation among many other things reveal themselves to the sadhaka. This is a situation that no scientist can ever fathom or reach with limited material equipment.

"After the Vishuddi Chakra the spark of light, now like the rising sun, explodes into brilliant light that pales a thousand suns as Kundalini reaches the Ajna Chakra, or the frontal wheel, located in between the eyebrows. This is a place of extreme bliss, divine love and peace. It is a state where there is the constant effulgence of the Lord. Many saints and prophets could be seen all immersed in the fathomless, infinite ocean of bliss, divine love and peace. Civilizations in distant galaxies and planets are seen in this and other dimensions, some in their infancy and some eons ahead of us, thriving well and evolving. Gods and goddesses are higher beings, so much more powerful and benevolent, who reveal themselves. This is beyond the symbolism. However, both are true.

"Going beyond the Ajna Chakra is the ultimate stage of Sahasrara, or the Crown Chakra, with a thousand petals where the individual soul becomes one with the Universal Soul, or the Paramatma, or the Lord. This is an incomprehensible state, which is beyond bliss and peace. This is the doorway to the actual spiritual world—a world of Divine Love and bliss that can be comprehended by divine souls only. This is Vaikuntha—where there is no vibration. Before Vaikuntha, the sadhaka can get the revelation of the Vishwarupa Darshan, or the vision of the Universal Self of the Lord, the vision that the Supreme Lord Krishna revealed to Arjuna at the battlefields of Kurukshetra more than five thousand years ago.

"After passing the Sahasrara Chakra, the Kundalini has to pass through different [24]eighteen Mahavidyas, or great wisdoms, which are energized subtle centers encircling the Sahasrara area. Finally, the Goddess Shakti unites with Shiva in an act termed as Maithuna Yoga in our earthly terms. This state beyond

[24] Śrī Kālī, Śrī Tārā, Śrīmātā Śōdasi, Mulprakriti Bhuvneshvarī,Chinnamasta,Bhairavi, Annapurna, Mahādurgā, Jayadurgā, Śrī Kamalā, Mātangi, Baglamukhi, Tvaritā, Sarasvatī, Nityā, Tripurāputā, Dhumavati and Śrī MahīśaMardini.

the [25]turiya state of extreme bliss is called Sat-Chit-Ananda (Pure Existence, Pure Wisdom, and Pure Bliss). That is the Supreme Lord. You become one with Brahman or Parabrahman or The Supreme Lord and become one with the entire existence. You realize the Oneness of the whole Creation.

"It is the experience of saints that in this world of spirituality, there is no distinction of race, religion, sex or any other material divisive forces. It is all light, colors, holy symbolism, OM and other holy sounds and visions of subtle existences of expansions of the Lord and of human beings beyond death, of creation at an infancy and creation at its best. The mysteries of creation get revealed slowly but surely. The human consciousness dissolves in the Universal Consciousness or Ultimate Reality. Humans are the universe themselves, only covered by material energy, for which they have forgotten their real identity. This process enables humans to realize their real identity. This creation is for all of us to experience life and its complexities and also experience divinity, which is the core.

"The saints have said in all the scriptures that the human being is the best creation of the Lord. It is a vehicle with which ultimate perfection can be attained. Even the demi-gods cannot attain that stage as they are assigned certain duties for which they are limited in their levels of realization."

It was a long talk and with minor breaks in between to snatch a samosa or a new cup of coffee. I looked at Madhu and he was too overwhelmed to speak.

He looked at me with emotions flooding his eyes and face. "Shomikda, How do you know so much about these secret sciences?"

"My friend, I have been blessed to have the association of God-realized saints from childhood. It is their knowledge, not mine. I am simply a messenger of their wisdom," I said humbly. "Madhu, tell me about the Brihadeeshwara Temple of Thanjavur, where you had visited also," I said.

Madhu smiled and spoke, [26]"Brihadeeshwara Temple (Peruvudaiyar Kovil) is a temple dedicated to Lord Shiva in Thanjavur in Tamil Nadu. It is also known as Periya Kovil, Rajarajeswara Temple and Rajarajesvaram. It is one of the largest temples in India and is an example of South Indian architecture during the Chola period. Built by Emperor Rajaraja Chola I and completed in 1010 A.D., the temple turned one thousand years old in 2010. The temple

[25] Three states of consciousness, namely waking (*jagrat*), dreaming (*svapna*), deep sleep (*suṣupti*), which are empirically experienced by human beings. Turiya is the fourth state beyond deep sleep.

[26] Source: Incredibleindia.org

is part of the UNESCO World Heritage Site known as the 'Great Living Chola Temples,' with the other two being the Gangaikonda Cholapuram and Airavatesvara temple.

"The temple stands amidst fortified walls that were probably added in the 16th century. The vimanam (temple tower) is 216 feet (66 meters) high and is the tallest in the world. The Kumbam (the apex or the bulbous structure on the top) of the temple is carved out of a single rock and weighs around eighty tons.

"There is a big statue of Nandi (sacred bull), carved out of a single rock measuring about 16 feet (4.9 meters) long and 13 feet (4.0 meters) high at the entrance. The entire temple structure is made out of granite, the nearest sources of which are about 60 kilometers to the west of temple. The temple is one of the most visited tourist attractions in Tamil Nadu.

Arulmozhivarman, a Tamil emperor who was popular as Rajaraja Chola I, laid out foundations of Brihadeeshwara Temple during 1002 C.E. It was first among other great building projects by Tamil Chola. A symmetrical and axial geometry rules layout of this temple. Brihadeeshwara Temple is first among all buildings that make use of granite fully and it finished within five years, from 1004 A.D. to 1009 A.D.

"The greatest of Chola emperors, Rajaraja I (985 A.D. -1012 A.D.), the son of Sundara Chola (Parantaka-II) and Vanavan Mahadevi, built this magnificent temple named Brihadeeshwara at Thanjavur, the capital of Chola dynasty.

"Rajaraja-I named this temple as Rajarajesvaram and the deity Lord Shiva in Linga form as Peruvudaiyar.The temple is also known in the deity's name as Peruvudaiyarkovil (in Tamil language).

"On the same axis stand Gopurams (temple gateways) of the early phase at the eastern center of the cloister and the brick wall. They are the sole entrance spots to the temple precincts.

"The Brihadeeshwara Temple is the best representative of orthodox South Indian temple architecture." Madhu ended his description of the great temple of Brihadeeshwara in Thanjavur.

The day was rolling into the evening twilight with the last embers of the sunlight streaming through the side of the drapes on the windows.

"I will see you tomorrow, Shomikda," Madhu said as he prepared to leave.

"Sure, most welcome," I said as I walked him to the door.

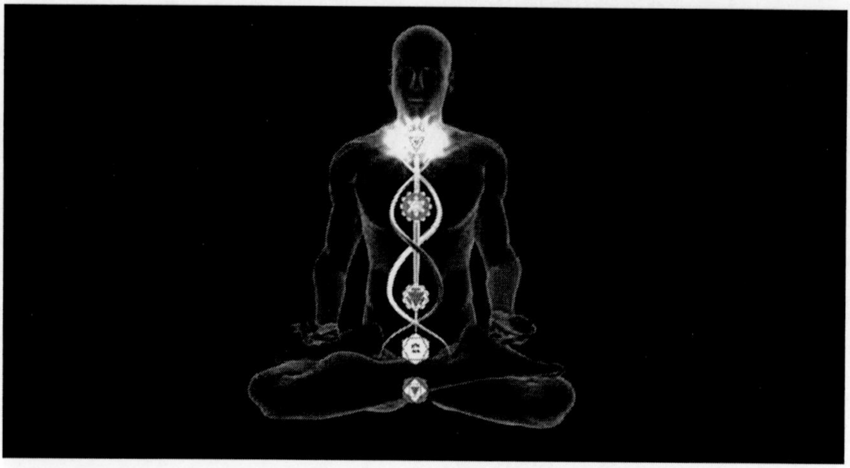

Silhouette in an enlightened Yoga meditation pose with five highlighted Chakras. Credit: 3000ad

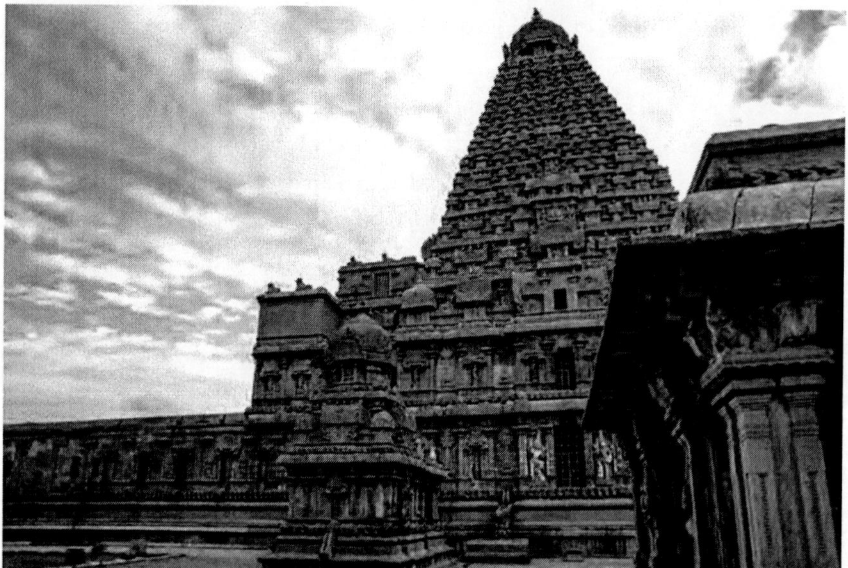

Great architecture of Hindu temple Brihadeshwara, located in Thanjavor, Tamil Nadu. Credit: a_lis

Chapter 6

The Spiritual World

The next day was a Sunday and Madhu called me in the morning requesting an audience with me to discuss the esoteric topics in more details. I, of course, agreed and my wife prepared some coffee, tea and some snacks to go with the coffee and tea.

At the appointed hour, Madhu rang the bell and greeted me and my wife as he swept into our living room wearing a coat as the chill had started to descend on Long Island, New York, already.

Madhu smiled at me and said, "Shomikda, I could not sleep properly yesterday thinking about the science behind our existence. Please tell me more. I am full of curiosity."

I said with a smile and a pause, collecting my thoughts and preparing to start my talk, "I will tell you about the spiritual world as seen by many saints, including Sarkarkaku.

"The Spiritual World and Creation

"The spark of light, or the Bindu of OM, that brings the sadhaka to the final stage of entry into the spiritual world has the living form of Lord Krishna in it. It is Lord Krishna who comes to take us from the bondage of the material creation to the spiritual world. He is depicted as dark blue in color as He reveals Himself fully in the region of dark blue color before Sahasrara. He is the Supreme Personality of Godhead who is beyond all creation and is the Cause of all Causes. He is the God whom everyone prays knowingly or unknowingly. He is the Paramatma or Parabrahman. He is the unmanifest and the manifest. He is beyond all understanding or comprehension. It is what Lord Chaitanya said, "Achinta Bhedabhed Tattwa" or the "Unthinkable Singularity-Duality Philosophy. In Indian philosophy and spirituality, we believe in One Supreme Brahman or Parabrahman manifested in countless forms.'

"In the Bhagavad Gita, Lord Krishna says that He is in everything in this Creation and everything or the whole Creation is in Him. He is beyond this Creation also. God Realization is to experience and see Lord Krishna or the Ultimate Reality in everything, everywhere, including oneself. Adwaita philosophy or Oneness of everything is a perfect reality that we need to realize. Everything is an expansion and manifestation of the Ultimate Reality. But the philosophies expressing a difference between Ultimate Reality and us are the initial steps toward the final realization of Oneness. We need to start from the lower rungs of duality and build a loving relationship with the Ultimate Reality in the form of the embodiment of Sat-Chid-Ananda, Lord Krishna or any other divine manifestation of the Lord. Through the combined austerity of Karma, Jyana, Dhyana and Bhakti Yogas and final surrender to Lord Krishna can we go toward realization of the Ultimate Reality and through the final removal of all illusion we can realize that there is nothing other than the Ultimate Reality. It is so beyond all expression and understanding that it can only be realized as the Oneness in Creation and beyond. But in Indian spiritual culture we respect everyone including the people following the dualities. Everyone is on the path of evolution and needs to follow the path suitable for him/her based on their level of spiritual evolution.

"There are descriptions in the Vedas about the various incarnations that the world would be blessed with. They are ten main incarnations and twenty-four secondary incarnations. It also states about the Supreme Lord Krishna's advent from whom all other incarnations emanate. A detail is already given about their advent, family, work and life. The ten incarnations include Matsya (Fish), Kurma (Tortoise), Varaha (Boar), Narasimha (Half-Man-Half-Lion), Vamana (Dwarf), Parasurama (Brahmin warrior), Rama, Balaram, Buddha and Kalki. However, there are incarnations of Lord Shiva, Lord Dattatreya, and other Gods and Goddesses, and there are siddhas, saints and other divine personalities.

[27]"The Vedic texts state that the Supreme Personality exists in the spiritual world prior to any creation as one without a second. By His Supreme Will the cosmic manifestation takes place. God is Supreme bliss or Pleasure, which is our true character as we have emerged from him. While Radharani takes the divine pleasure manifestation of the Lord, Lord Balaram is the predominator of the creative energy.

"The creation of the material world takes place through many steps. An expansion of the Lord, known as an incarnation, makes the first step toward creation—Maha Vishnu, the master of eternal time, space, cause and effects, mind, elements and all living beings. From Maha Vishnu comes the infinite expanse of Causal Ocean, where He lies down accompanied by all the ingredients of material creation, or Maya. This is the border of the material world and the spiritual world.

"Maha Vishnu enters into Yoga Nidra, or a divine sleep, and dreams the creation, maintenance, and annihilation of the cosmic manifestation. The divine sleep proves that whole creation happened through consciousness. The Holy Trinity of Lord Brahma, Lord Vishnu and Lord Shiva are all expressions of cosmic consciousness, depicted with Maha Vishnu's dream. It is from this Cosmic Consciousness that the whole Creation emerges. It creates, maintains and dissolves everything onto itself. Saints say that the present creation is the 84th of a cycle of creation, sustenance and dissolution. It will continue till 112 times and then it will be only energy.

"Mahamaya, the material energy, causes the material creation and also has the total material ingredients in its nonmanifest form from consciousness.

"Then, with the interactions of the time factor, the total ingredients of matter, called mahat-tattva, become manifest and gradually creation takes place. The Supreme Being creates infinite number of universes like atoms with a combination of water, air, fire, sky, ego and mahat-tattva surrounded by pradhana or the unmanifest material energy in the form of Causal Ocean. The universes are created with the exhalation of Maha Vishnu and return to His Body with inhalation.

"After creation of the universe, Maha Vishnu expands himself into infinite forms as Garbhodakashayi Vishnu and enters each universe. From Garbhodakashayi Vishnu's body an expanse of water (not the water that we know it to be) called the Garbodaka Ocean is formed and fills half the universe. He again lies down in a slumber on that ocean and when the desire for activity begins,

[27] Srimad Bhagavatam.

the total form of all fruitive activities and living entities pierces through Sri Vishnu's abdomen in the form of a lotus. This lotus forms the heavenly planet that gives birth to the self-born Lord Brahma, the personality of Vedic wisdom. Then Sri Vishnu also expands into infinite expansions known as Ksirodaka-shayi Vishnu and this becomes the Supersoul within every living entity. Symbolism and reality both exist simultaneously in different lokas, or dimensions. "The Shivalinga that we worship is the 'Golden Egg' that was a precursor to the creation or expansion as explained in the Rig Veda.

"Lord Brahma engineers the second level of creation by creating the material worlds and the living entities within them. He also creates the demigods and the gandharvas, apsaras or angels, siddhas and other astral beings.

"This wisdom, enshrined in the Vedas, is passed from Lord Brahma to the first perfect man on this earth as also in other planets.

"The process of creation from the subtle form to the material level takes 51 quantum vibrations. These 51 vibrations form the 51 alphabets of the Sanskrit language. It is the mother of all languages and is the divine language that has come from the stages of creation to its material form. When the creation manifested itself into the material form, it was represented by the word OM. It manifested itself from the subtle-most level to the material level as the 'Word of God,' which is God. It is because of the divine origin and the part of Creation, Sanskrit language today has been accepted by some scientific groups as the most scientific language in the world. Furthermore, it is a very potent language with each syllable having tremendous potential energy. If rendered properly, it can give results like nothing else.

"The symbolism of the material creation is represented in the image of Mother Kali. The figure of Shiva represents the inert state from which all creation arose. Mother Kali has a necklace having fifty heads strung together. These represent the fifty quantum vibrations and the 51st one in her hand represents the creation of the material world. She is dark colored as she is beyond all comprehension and is unclothed as she cannot be limited by anything. Her tongue that sticks out is because of the yogic mudra, or gestures, that happen to sadhakas naturally when they reach a very highly elevated stage where Mother Kali reveals Herself (it can go in the throat or stick out).

"Similarly, Mother Durga is Nature, who represents balance in the Cosmos. She controls or annihilates forces that have gone against the Cosmic Laws to bring the eternal balance in Nature or Creation. That is why She receives weapons from all the forces of Nature. Mahisasura is something in the creation that has gone awry. Mother Durga uses the

[28]trishula with the three qualities of sattwa, rajas, and tamas to stop it or end it.

"Sadhana is something that should be done at all times to uplift ourselves. We should offer everything that we do as an offering to God. Then it is the best that we have to offer, it is full of devotion and it is pure. That is the best way we should lead our lives. We should remember that God is our eternal friend, relation, everything. We should develop a relationship with Him. Then our lives will be satisfying, blissful, successful and contributive to the good of the society.

"The Supreme Personality of Godhead

"It is through the infinite mercy of the Supreme Lord that He reveals Himself to us through His Divine incarnations. The Vedas define the Supreme Lord as Sat (Absolute Truth), Chit (Pure Consciousness) and Ananda (Pure bliss).

* [29]"In the present Dwapara Yuga, Lord Krishna, the Supreme Lord in totality, took birth to play His divine pastimes for His devotees to see, listen and mediate on. Due to its omnipresent, omnipotent and omniscient nature, the Supreme Lord can project or manifest itself as a human being. It is once in twenty-eight Kalpas (very long periods of time) that the Supreme Lord incarnates Himself to play the divine role. The Vedas and the Brahma Samhitas proclaim the advent and the Absolute Divinity of Lord Krishna in innumerous stanzas. One of them is a verse from the Brahma Samhita:

ishvarah paramah krishnah
sac-cid-ananda-vigrahaha
anadir adir govindaha
sarva-karana-karanam

"(Krishna, who is known as Govinda, is the Supreme Personality of Godhead. He has an eternal blissful spiritual body. He is the Origin of all. He has no other origin and He is the Prime Cause of all causes.)

***"The Atharva Vediya Gopalatapani Upanishad, Purva Vibhaga, verse 36, states:**

om namo vishva-rupaya
vishva-sthity-anta-hetave
vishveshvaraya vishvaya
govindaya namo namaha

---

[28] Trident used by Lord Shiva with the three extensions on top.

[29] *Krishna.com.*

"(Lord Brahma, speaking to the great sages and saints, prayed to Lord Krishna as follows: 'I offer my humble obeisances to Lord Krishna, who is the giver of pleasure to the cows, whose external form is the form of the universe, who is the cause of the maintenance and dissolution of the material universe, and who is the Lord of the universe.')

*"Sri Krishna is the source of all other incarnations and forms of God. He is the ultimate and end of all Truth and philosophical enquiry, the goal or end result of Vedanta. He is the all-attractive personality and source of all pleasure for which we are always hankering. He is the origin from which everything else manifests. He is the unlimited source of all power, wealth, fame, beauty, wisdom, and renunciation. Thus, no one is greater than Him. Since Lord Krishna is the source of all living beings, He is also considered the Supreme Father and source of all worlds.

*"The *Brihadaranyaka Upanishad* says, *purnam idam purnat purnam udacyate*: 'Although He expands in many ways, He keeps His original personality. His original spiritual body remains as it is.' Thus, we can understand that God can expand His energies in many ways but is not affected or diminished in His potency.

*"The *Svetasvatara Upanishad* (6.6) also states: 'The Supreme Personality of Godhead, the original person, has multifarious energies. He is the origin of material creation, and it is due to Him only that everything changes. He is the protector of religion and annihilator of all sinful activities. He is the master of all opulence.'

*[30]"Other verses that describe the nature and characteristics of the Supreme Being are related by Lord Krishna Himself in the *Bhagavad-gita*, such as: 'I am the father of the universe, the mother, the support and the grandsire. I am the object of knowledge, the purifier and the syllable *OM*. I am also the *Rig*, the *Sama* and the *Yajur Vedas*. I am the goal, the sustainer, the master, the witness, the abode, the refuge and the most dear friend. I am the creation and

[30] Bhagavad Gita As It Is.

the annihilation, the basis of everything, the resting place and the eternal seed' (*Bg*. 9:17-18).

*'"I am the source of all spiritual and material worlds. Everything emanates from Me. The wise, who perfectly know this, engage in my worship with all their hearts' (*Bg*.10:8).

*"Arjuna said: 'You are the Supreme Personality of Godhead, the ultimate abode, the purest, the Absolute Truth. You are the eternal, transcendental, original person, the unborn, the greatest. All the great sages such as Narada, Asita, Devala and Vyasa confirm this truth about You, and now You Yourself are declaring it to me' (*Bg*.10:12-13).

*'"Know that all opulent, beautiful and glorious creations spring from but a spark of My splendor. But what need is there, Arjuna, for all this detailed knowledge? With a single fragment of Myself I pervade and support this entire universe' (*Bg*.10:41-42).

*"O conqueror of wealth, there is no truth superior to Me. Everything rests upon Me, as pearls are strung on a thread.

*"O son of Kunti, I am the taste of water, the light of the sun and the moon, the syllable OM in the Vedic mantras; I am the sound in ether and ability in man.

*"I am the original fragrance of the earth, and I am the heat in fire. I am the life of all that lives, and I am the austerities of all ascetics.

*"O son of Prtha, know that I am the original seed of all existences, the intelligence of the intelligent, and the prowess of all-powerful men.

*"The whole cosmic order is under Me. Under My will it is automatically manifested again and again, and under My will it is annihilated at the end.

*"I am the goal, the sustainer, the master, the witness, the abode, the refuge, and the most dear friend. I am the creation and the annihilation, the basis of everything, the resting place and the eternal seed.

*"Of all creations I am the beginning and the end and also the middle, O Arjuna. Of all sciences I am the spiritual science of the self, and among logicians I am the conclusive truth.

*"Arjuna saw in that universal form unlimited mouths, unlimited eyes, unlimited wonderful visions. The form was decorated with many celestial ornaments and bore many divine upraised weapons. He wore celestial garlands and

garments, and many divine scents were smeared over His body. All was wondrous, brilliant, unlimited, all-expanding. If hundreds of thousands of suns were to rise at once into the sky, their radiance might resemble the effulgence of the Supreme Person in that universal form. If hundreds of thousands of suns were to rise at once into the sky, their radiance might resemble the effulgence of the Supreme Person in that universal form.

*"Arjuna said: 'My dear Lord Krishna, I see assembled in Your body all the demigods and various other living entities. I see Brahma sitting on the lotus flower, as well as Lord Shiva and all the sages and divine serpents. All the various manifestations of Lord Shiva, the Adityas, the Vasus, the Sadhyas, the Visvedevas, the two Asvis, the Maruts, the forefathers, the Gandharvas, the Yaksas, the Asuras and the perfected demigods are beholding You in wonder.

*"I am seated in everyone's heart, and from Me come remembrance, knowledge and forgetfulness. By all the Vedas, I am to be known. Indeed, I am the compiler of Vedanta, and I am the knower of the Vedas.

*"Because I am transcendental, beyond both the fallible and the infallible, and because I am the greatest, I am celebrated both in the world and in the Vedas as that Supreme Person.

*"Whoever knows Me as the Supreme Personality of Godhead, without doubting, is the knower of everything. He therefore engages himself in full surrender to Me, O son of Bharata.

*"This is the most confidential part of the Vedic scriptures, O sinless one, and it is disclosed now by Me. Whoever understands this will become wise, and his endeavors will know perfection.

"The Purpose of Life

"The purpose of life is self-realization and the reestablishment of our lost relationship with the Supreme Personality of Godhead. According to the Vedic traditions, the perfection of life is to realize one's relationship with Krishna, or God, and serve Him with all our heart and soul. Of course, the nature of our service may take different forms, but the essence would be the same.

"The Vedic scriptures lay down the steps that enable a person to elevate himself to the level of a realized soul. This is propounded in the Hata Yoga for the control of the body, breath and the nerves. Raja Yoga helps in the mastery over the mind. This is a part of Astanga Yoga, or the eight disciplines. They are:

Yama-moral and ethical disciplines of non-injury, truthfulness, non-stealing, continence and non-covetousness;

Niyama-constitutes religious or spiritual observances including purity of body, speech and mind; contentment; austerities; study of scriptures for self-knowledge; devotion and surrender to God;

Asana-steady and relaxed postures;

Pranayama-regulation and control of breathing;

Pratyahara-withdrawal of senses from sense objects;

Dharana-concentration;

Dhyana-meditation;

Samadhi-super-conscious state

"With perfection in Hata Yoga and Raja Yoga, the sadhaka can do his duties better or the Yoga of Work (Karma Yoga) becomes better. He can do all that he is supposed to do to the best of his ability without attaching himself to the fruit of the action. With renunciation in the fruits of all actions, knowledge and wisdom rise in him and the study and contemplation of the scriptures helps him to attain perfection in the Yoga of Knowledge (Jyana Yoga). With knowledge, understanding, practices and devotion, he is able to concentrate better in meditation and he attains perfection in the Yoga of Meditation (Dhyana Yoga). Perfection in the Yoga of Meditation develops with a deep devotion to the Lord (Bhakti Yoga). Devotion overflows in the practitioner and he attains the mercy of the Lord and self-realization. This is called Kriya Yoga, which is a combination of all the yogas. This was taught by Lord Krishna to Arjuna in the Gita.

"But the Vedic scriptures do not denounce opulence in life. It has divided life into four parts: Brahmacharya, or the period of learning, self-development, abstinence and austerities; Grihastya — raising a good family with good values and virtues, providing for the family in the best possible way with the roots firmly entrenched in spirituality and raising good children for the good of the society; Vanaprasthya — the period of slow renunciation after the children settle down and become independent; Sanyasa — absolute renunciation and totally immersed in the sadhana of the Lord.

"It has also propounded that a human being should follow Dharma, or righteousness; accrue Artha or wealth in a righteous way; enjoy Kama or enjoy life in a righteous manner; and strive to attain Moksha or liberation as the ultimate goal of life.

"Hence, it is plain from here that the Vedic scriptures do ask us to lead a balanced life without sacrificing everything to fulfill any one aspect of life.

"Spiritual practices lead to flowering of divine qualities, including fearlessness, purification of one's existence, cultivation of spiritual knowledge, charity, self-control, study of the Vedas, austerity, simplicity, nonviolence, truthfulness, freedom from anger, renunciation, tranquility, aversion to faultfinding, compassion for all living entities, freedom from covetousness, gentleness, modesty, steady determination, vigor, forgiveness, fortitude, cleanliness, and freedom from envy and from the passion for honor.

"Wisdom of the scriptures and the sages emanate from within us as we continue in the upliftment of our consciousness through our sadhana.

"It is desire, lust, anger, greed, jealousy, and ego that give rise to all pain and suffering. We must remove all these vices from our inside to attain peace and happiness.

"The nations today are seeped in these vices created due to ignorance of spiritual knowledge or wisdom that was once prevalent all over the world. They have failed to see the thread of commonality that binds us all, and that our eternal nature is peace, happiness, love and harmony. Unless the leaders of nations are trained in the science, there would be continuing bloodshed and annihilation of races and civilizations through the history of humanity.

"Each one of the wise ones, who share this wisdom, should play an active role in disseminating the knowledge of harmony and peace and guide the world away from self-destruction toward peace, unity, prosperity, happiness and development. The banner should read help and not fight, assimilation and not destruction, harmony and peace and not dissention.

"Can we make the world turn around? It is up to each one of us to exemplify and be a role model; spread our areas of influence beyond our family, friends and immediate society; and embrace humanity at large and show them that the path of happiness lies in international brotherhood, in harmony, in true spirituality and not in violent dismembering. The best way to develop a strong value base is through spiritual practices and the more we do it with intensity and devotion, the more would our pots become full.

"The above traits of human character should be imbibed from childhood. The parents should exemplify and show the children the right values and principles. They should encourage children to develop the love of God and not I paused for a sip of coffee and a handful of snacks as I lay back on the sofa to rest after a long talk.

Madhu was overwhelmed to hear of my talk on the spiritual world. He slowly recollected himself from his trance-like stupor and said that he had also visited the Nataraja Temple at Chidambaram in Tamil Nadu. It is one of five holiest shrines dedicated to Lord Shiva, and as in each Lord Shiva is represented here as one of the five elements of material world, here being space.

[31]"The temple is over two millennia old. It has been patronized by theSouth Indian dynasties. Their donations have enriched the temple and carved thousands of inscriptions on its walls.

"The temple has eleven shrines, five halls or sabhas and the sacred water tank, Sivaganga and nine gateways, or gopurams. The largest sabha, known as the Raja Sabha, is located on the east of the water tank. It has one thousand pillars representing the Sahashrara Chakra. The remaining four halls are located in the innermost sacred courtyard, nrtiya sabha, which is a 56-pillared dance hall. Deva sabha houses the images of Lord Shiva's family members and administrative meetings of the temple are held here. The most important sabhas are the chit sabha (house of consciousness) and kanaka sabha, which form an important part of the temple.

In the golden sanctum of the chit sabha, Lord Shiva is represented by anthropomorphic form as Nataraja performing the Ananda Tandava dance of bliss. The other forms are a crystal lingam and as formless empty space represented with a garland of 51 hanging golden leaves.

"Nataraja represents panchakritya, or five functions of the godhead, such as creation, preservation, destruction, embodiment and salvation. He is manifestation of the primal rhythmic cosmic energy.

"In the Nataraja statue the demon under Lord Shiva's feet signifies crushing of our egos and the darkness of ignorance. The fire in his hand signifies the power of destruction of evil.

---

[31] Ref: Temples of India, Abode of the Divine, Tarun Chopra, Prakash Books. Printed and bound at Thomson Press, 2018, pp. 244-251.

"The raised hand represents that He is the savior of all life forms.

"The arc of fire represents the continuous creation and destruction of the cosmos.

"The drum in His hand represents the origin of life forms and time.

"The lotus pedestal represents OM, or the primordial sound.

"His right eye, left eye and third eye represent the sun, moon and knowledge, respectively.

"His right earring (makara kundalam) and left earring (sthri kundalam) represent non-duality, the union of man (right) and woman (left).

"The crescent moon in His hair represents benevolence and beauty. "The flowing River Ganga, through his matted hair, represents eternity of life.

"The dreading of His hair represents the force of His dance."

Madhau paused and continued, "Shomikda, it is amazing to learn about our tradition, culture, and treasures that made us the world leaders in the distant past. We need to reclaim it as we help humanity to come up and be happy, not an isolated nation of any groups."

We had lunch together partaking the delicious meal that my wife had prepared.

While having lunch, Madhu turned toward me and said, "Shomikda, how would you trust the visions that Sarkarkaku described?"

I said, "Sarkarkaku said various things about us and many people through his visions, which all came true, and I also had the experience of the visions that he described in the initial stages. So, I know that I am on a similar path too. But most important is the fact and understanding that some people have the capacity to see beyond our material world through austerities. There is an infinite world beyond our material understanding and knowledge. What I stated was his experience. Others may have different experiences. It just explains the infinite possibilities and capabilities that every human being has. You only have to arouse your inner immense energy to raise your consciousness to transform your life into Life Divine."

After settling down on the sofa once again, we restarted our conversation.

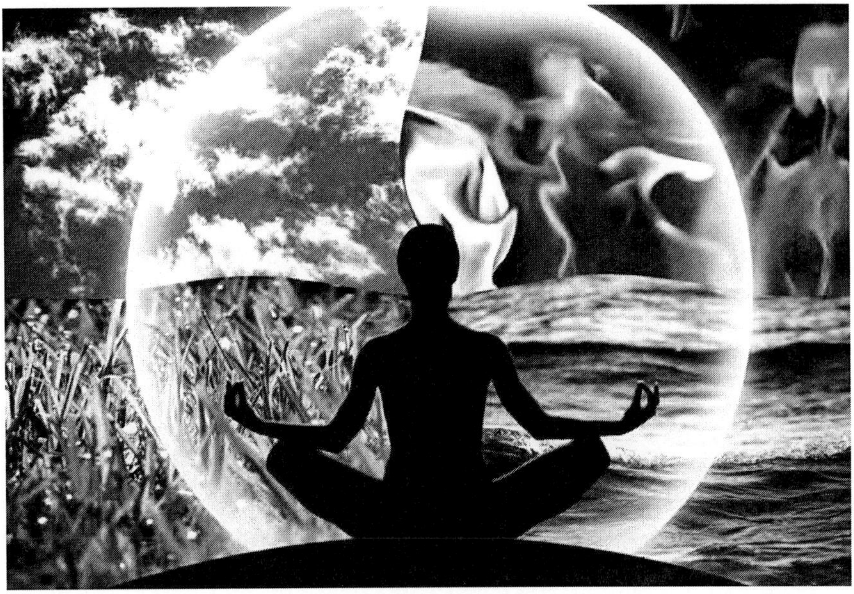

Female yoga figure in a transparent sphere, composed of five natural elements (water, fire, earth, air, space) as a concept for controlling emotions and power over nature. Credit: Zuberka

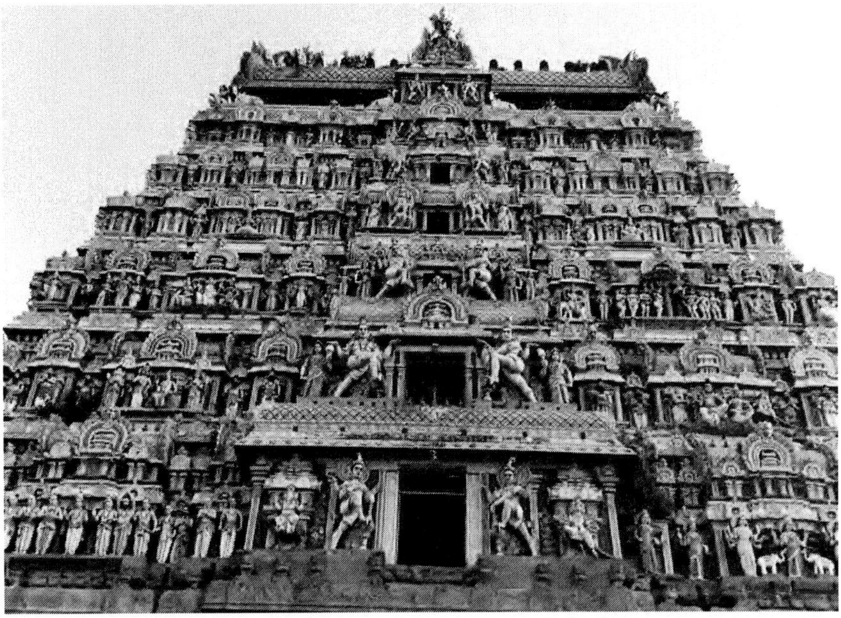

The main gopuram of Chidambaram Nataraja temple or Thillai Nataraja Temple in Chidambaram, Tamil Nadu. Credit: Kruthi R

Chapter 7

Searching for Happiness

Madhu and I met the following weekend at our place. While settling with our cups of hot coffee in the midst of a wintery mix blowing through the island, we commenced our conversations on human existence.

"Let me talk about an intrinsic quality that we all possess—Happiness," I started the conversation eagerly.

[32]"When alive, physical (adhibhautik), divine (adhidaivik) and spiritual (adhyatmik) are the types of happiness according to the scriptures. These types are classified according to the cause of happiness or unhappiness.

1. **Physical (adhibhautik):** As an example, the sun being of the form of radiance has extreme heat. The warm sunlight feels pleasant in winter but the same proves painful during summer. Thus, the happiness or unhappiness experienced from the various objects created from the five great cosmic elements (panchmahabhuta) are termed as physical (adibhautik). The happiness and unhappiness from fire, drought, excessive rainfall, so also from animals and man are included in this type.
2. **Divine (adhidaivik):** The deity Savita controls all the activities of the sun. This deity is appeased by one who repeats (chants) Her Name and blesses him. Hence, such happiness is termed as divine (adhidaivik) happiness. However, should this deity get angry, it curses the person who consequently has to experience unhappiness. In short, the happiness and unhappiness arising from the grace of the deities or

[32] *Spirituality*, published by Sanatan Sanstha.

their rage, those from ghosts, spirits, etc., unhappiness experienced after death are included in this category.

3. **Spiritual (adhyatmik):**
   Physical: Due to an imbalance of the three doshas—vata (wind), pitta (bile) and kapha (phlegm).
   Psychological: Due to the six vices (shadripu), namely, desire (kam), anger (krodh), greed (lobh), vanity (mada), attachment (moha) and jealousy (matsar). These vices too are dependent on the three doshas—vata, pitta and kapha.

To overcome the unhappiness arising from physical and divine causes, generally external measures need to be employed. Thus, this unhappiness is curable with external remedies. Psychological unhappiness, on the other hand, needs internal measures for their amelioration.

"After death people experience unhappiness on not obtaining those objects that gave oneself happiness when alive.

A. Worldly: Relative to objects
B. In the subtle worlds: Relative to objects
C. Spiritual: Not relative to objects

"A relative experience:

A. Relative to unhappiness: People feel happy after recovering from an illness. If one who is unhappy due to ignorance is enlightened with knowledge the unhappiness gets removed; this can be called happiness relative to unhappiness.
B. Relative to happiness: When a well-to-do person procures a huge fortune, he feels happier. If the reverse is true, one gets unhappiness relative to happiness and unhappiness.

"Individual (vyashti) and for the sake of society (samashti)

"Like every individual the aim of the society too should be happiness. Happiness of the society is the happiness of all or most of its members. Despite keeping this as the objective, society has to remain content with psychological happiness. With respect to physical happiness, it is seen that if an individual begins experiencing excessive happiness, he begins to encroach on the happiness of another. Food, clothing and shelter are the basic needs of man. But it is not possible for society to provide them in abundance to the entire population. It is assumed that every individual will be given a minimal share of food. However, if one tries to acquire an extra portion, another is deprived of it. Psychological happiness differs in this aspect. As an individual begins to experience more and more psychological happiness, he becomes the cause for others' happiness, for instance by giving wonderful dance and vocal recitals, etc. Consequently, others too, acquire happiness from all this and as a result the artists become famous. Fame is a very luring psychological happiness. Just like sandalwood, which imparts its fragrance to others, by reducing one's physical happiness man should sacrifice oneself for the sake of others and be praised by society. This proves to be favorable for both and so the society too makes progress.

"Happiness is of three types: Sattvik (mostly Sattvik), Rajasic (mostly Rajasic) and Tamasic (mostly Tamasic).

A. **Sattvik:** Giving happiness to others without thinking about one's own happiness or suffering. Giving happiness to others does not reduce one's happiness, as actually it is 100% happiness. This is happiness arising from the mind.

B. **Rajasik:** Trying to acquire happiness without causing any unhappiness to others. The happiness obtained from the sense organs and the motor organs is called rajasik happiness, e.g., eating a delicacy. In this instance, happiness or contentment is obtained instantly but ultimately it culminates into unhappiness for the reasons given below.

   1. One cannot experience a lot of happiness, e.g., one can get a stomach upset by overeating a rich, spicy dish.
   2. One cannot get the objects the moment they are desired, e.g., the sweet shop may be closed or a particular sweet may not be available in the shop.
   3. Sometimes it so happens that the happiness gets converted into a necessity, e.g., after enjoying talking on the mobile phone it becomes a habit. Thereafter, if the phone is unavailable for even a day, one feels miserable.

C. **Tamasik:** One derives happiness by inflicting others with unhappiness and running away from the hardships of life, e.g., drinking alcohol, taking narcotics, harassing others. This may also be termed as happiness arising from ignorance.

"Generally, happiness experienced by the intellect is sattvik, that by the mind is rajasik and that by the body is tamasik in nature. The happiness derived after the intellect acquires spiritual knowledge is merely due to the elimination of ignorance, which is gross. When the mind experiences happiness, its grossness too is decreased.

"A pleasurable feeling, a pleasurable sensation (mod) and happiness (pramod)

"When a person sees an object that endows happiness, a pleasurable feeling is generated in the mind. When that object is procured there is a pleasurable sensation, and when experiencing it there is happiness.

"According to the organs...

"All types of happiness arise from Brahman (God principle):

A. **Brahmanand (Advaitanand):** Happiness in its pure form is termed as Brahmanand, or (Advaitanand), i.e., bliss arising from Brahman or non-duality (advait).
B. **Vidyanand (dnyananand):** Happiness obtained from the intellect is termed as vidyanand, or dnyananand, i.e., happiness obtained from knowledge (dhyana).
C. **Vasananand:** Happiness obtained from gratification of desires and aspirations, so also of anger, egoism, jealousy, etc., is termed as vasananand, i.e., happiness obtained from desire (vasana).
D. **Vishayanand:** Happiness (worldly happiness or object pleasure) obtained from the sense organs is termed as vishayanand.

"Happiness other than bliss obtained from Brahman (Brahmanand) is of an impure nature and cannot grant complete contentment. Although all types of happiness arise from Brahman (God principle), the quality of happiness depends on the purity of the person experiencing it. Just as a reflection of an object is clearly seen in clean water but is not at all seen in muddy water, similarly only if the ego (aham) is pure does one experience the supreme bliss of Brahman and not otherwise.

"Peak of happiness

"The peak of happiness is orgasm and that of unhappiness is when a seeker gets dejected when he does not find God. Since the happiness obtained during intercourse is physical, it is tamasik in nature, while the unhappiness experienced by the seeker is sattvik.

"That which causes grief, stress, unhappiness or pain has to be sacrificed even though it may be an organ of our body" – **Mahabharata 12.174.43.**

"Instead of trying to acquire happiness, man makes more efforts to reduce suffering, for example by going to a doctor when ill, getting the radio or car repaired when it breaks down, etc. Very few people regularly exercise to remain healthy, get the car serviced periodically, etc. The efforts made to alleviate suffering are not always successful. For instance, an incurable illness, old age and death are things about which an ordinary person can do nothing to reduce the consequent suffering.

"In short, since one does not know how to obtain bliss, the life of the majority of people is spent in trying to find small pleasures and in overcoming unhappiness.

"Qualities of happiness

> "The hair on the body, tips of the nails, sweat and faeces do not experience unhappiness."
>
> **–Charak Sharir 1**

"Happiness obtained through the physical body through the medium of the five senses

"Eating one's favorite dish, listening to music, watching a game, etc., are pleasurable initially but if one repeats the act over and over again the happiness obtained from it goes on decreasing and ultimately the same thing causes unhappiness. Hence in the Shrimad Bhagvadgita (2:14), it is said, 'Cool and warm responses of the sense organs with objects give happiness or unhappiness, respectively.'

"If a person begins eating a favorite dessert like cake, then he will relish the first three or four plates. He will eat the next three or four plates with less enthusiasm and finally will refuse more. If he is forced to eat it, then it will make him unhappy. The same occurs if one listens to the same song or watches the same movie over and over again. That is why the holy text Adhyatmaramayan teaches that ultimately every kind of happiness culminates in unhappiness.

"Happiness obtained through the subtle body (desire body, mental body)
"The quality and quantity of happiness obtained by the mind, for example by loving someone, is higher than that obtained through the five senses. Its duration is also longer. Later when love successfully culminates in marriage, the happiness obtained from it decreases.

"Happiness obtained through the causal body (intellect)
"Although the happiness obtained by the intellect by studying a particular subject, understanding it, solving a difficult mathematical problem, discovering something after doing research, etc., is of a higher quality and quantity than the happiness obtained through the mind, that too is transitory.

"But beyond all these levels of sources of happiness is spiritual bliss. God is essentially bliss and it is the core of our beings. By doing penance and uplifting our consciousness, we are able to go inward to the depth of our souls, which is bliss. So, we have observed that highly realized souls are always happy in any situation or circumstance. That is the fundamental source of sustainable happiness and is infinite, eternal and all-encompassing."

I ended my talk and took another sip of a refilled cup of coffee and looked at Madhu, who looked at me with mesmerized eyes, drinking every word that I had said.

I broke his trance-like situation and asked him, "Madhu, tell me something about the temples of Mahabalipuram, where you had visited."

Collecting himself from his self-induced trance, Madhu took another sip at the coffee cup and started, "I had been to Mahabalipuram, an amazing place also known as the city of the Seven Pagodas by the British.

[33]"The Group of Monuments at Mahabalipuram is a collection of 7th- and 8th-century C.E. religious monuments in the coastal resort town of Mahabalipuram, Tamil Nadu, India is a UNESCO World Heritage Site. It is on the Coromandel Coast of the Bay of Bengal, 37 miles south of Chennai. The site has forty ancient monuments and temples, including one of the largest

---

[33] *IncredibleIndia.org.*

open-air rock reliefs in the world: the *Descent of the Ganges,* or *Arjuna's Penance.* The group contains several categories of monuments: *ratha* temples with monolithic processional chariots, built between 630 and 668 A.D.; *mandapa viharas* (cave temples) with narratives from the *Mahabharata* and Shaivite, Shakti or Shaaktha and Vaishnava inscriptions in a number of Indian languages and scripts; rock reliefs (particularly bas-reliefs); stone-cut temples built between 695 and 722 A.D., and archaeological excavations dated to the 6th century and earlier.

"The monuments were built during the Pallava dynasty. Known as the Seven Pagodas in many colonial-era publications, they are also called the Mamallapuram temples, or Mahabalipuram temples in contemporary literature. The site, restored after 1960, has been managed by the Archaeological Survey of India.

"Ratha

"The *ratha* temples, in Southern Mahabalipuram, are carved in the shape of chariots. Their artists used naturally occurring blocks of diorite and granite in sand, carving legends in stone. The best-known are the five monolithic structures projecting above the beach, known as the Five Rathas, or the Pandava Rathas. In the *Mahabharata,* the Pandavas are five brothers with a common wife, Draupadi. Although the symbolism and grouping of the temples have led to these popular names, they are neither true *rathas* nor dedicated to the Pandavas; they are temples dedicated to deities and concepts of the Shaivi, (Shiva), Vaishnavi (Vishnu) and Shakti (Durga) traditions of Hinduism. These *rathas* are dated to the 7th century.

"The Dharmaraja ratha has a square floor plan within a rectangular frame (26.75 feet x 20.67 feet) and is 35.67 feet high. It has an open porch supported by pillars. The temple's pyramidal tower consists of a vimana of shrinking squares, capped by an octagonal shikhara. Its pillars have seated lions at the base. It has three levels; the lowest is solid (probably never carved out), and the upper two have shrines. The two upper levels are connected by stairs carved into the stone. The middle level has two shrines, and the uppermost has one. The *ratha* walls have carvings and inscriptions. The western side of the top story has a Somaskanda image. The entablature integrates the secular with the divine, where human faces peek out of the *kudu* arches of the chariot. An Amaravati motif is carved below the cornice.

"Bhima Ratha (next to the Dharmaraja Ratha) is massive and has a roof resembling a vaulted barrel, reminiscent of woodwork. The *ratha* is 46 feet (14 meters) long, about 25 feet (7.6 meters) high and about 25 feet wide. Its incomplete interior was probably intended to house a reclining Vishnu (*anantasayana*). Unlike the other *rathas*, the temple has no inscriptions or sculptures. Its vimana is intricately carved on both sides of the roof. The cornice has seven pairs of kudus (Sanskrit: *gavaksha*). Above it are alternating *salas* and *kutas*, forming thirteen small vimanas. Above this layer are five *grivas* (necks, clerestory) carved into the shrine, like a niche flanked by small pilasters. The two on each side are the same size, and the middle one is larger. There is structural evidence on the top of eighteen original *kalashas* and two tridents.

"Arjuna Ratha, adjacent to Bhima Ratha, is also incomplete. One of the larger monuments, it is about six times smaller in area than the Dharmaraja Ratha. The square, two-level *ratha* has one shrine and mirrors the Dharmaraja Ratha; the decoration and structure of the cornice, kudus and *haras* are similar. However, its shikhara is hexagonal. The walls of the *ratha* are carved into panels with fourteen sculptures. Four are dvarapalas (Vishnu, a rishi with a student, Kartikeya—or Indra—and Shiva with Nandi), and the rest are humans at various stages of life. Arjuna Ratha has a lion and Nandi on each side between it and the adjacent Draupadi Ratha, but their orientation suggests that the *ratha* was not dedicated to Shiva. It may have been dedicated to Lord Ayyappan.

"The Draupadi Ratha is an 11-by-11-foot (3.4-by-3.4-meter) stone structure north of Arjuna Ratha, and they share a platform. It resembles a wooden hut and has a curved roof. There is a carved structure with alternating lions and elephants, and the shrine deity is missing. Its design is a simplified Nagara-style Hindu temple. The *ratha* has reliefs of Durga; three images are on the outer walls, and one is on an interior wall. The east-facing Durga is her Mahishasuramardini form, with the head of buffalo. Depicted elsewhere with her are devotees, *makaras* (mythical sea creatures) and *ganas* (mythical, comic dwarfs).

"The unfinished Nakula Sahadeva Ratha is an apsidal temple, a relatively uncommon Hindu design found in Aihole and elsewhere in India. The two-story, Vesara-style temple is 16 feet (4.9 meters) high and 18 feet (5.5 meters) long. It has *kutas* and *salas* style aedicule like the others but is unique in also having *panjaras* (an apsidal aedicule). The deity to whom it may have been dedicated is theorized to be Kartikeya, Brahma, Ayyappan or Indra. Northeast of the *ratha* are a standing elephant and Arjuna Ratha. Other *ratha* monuments at Mahabalipuram include the late-7th Century Ganesha Ratha, attributed to Parameshvara-varman I (grandson of Mahamalla).

"Cave Temples

"'Mandapa' is a Sanskrit term for a typically square vestibule, pillared hall or pavilion. It was a space for people to gather socially, usually for ceremonies and rite-of-passage rituals. Cells or sanctums would often be included, creating a *vihara*. Mandapas also refer to rock-cut cave temples or shrines, built according to the same concept, and Mamallapuram has many mandapas dated to the 7th and 8th centuries.

"The Varaha cave was excavated from a vertical wall on the west face of the main Mamallapuram hill. Its architecture is simple; a Vaishnavism-related cave temple, it is known for its four sculptures depicting Hindu legends: the Vamana-Trivikrama legend, the Varaha legend, the Durga legend and the Gajalakshmi legend. Srinivasan and other scholars date it to the 7th century.

"Kotikal

"Kotikal is a simple, early excavation with two pilasters on its facade. In front of it are sockets, suggesting a structural *mukhamandapa* (main hall). Inside the Kotikal cave temple are an oblong *ardha-mandapa* (half or partial hall) and a square sanctum (*garbha griya*). The front of the sanctum has mouldings and features similar to a free-standing temple.

"Dharmaraja cave temple entrance

"The Dharmaraja cave temple, also known as the Atyantakama cave temple, is on the south side of Mamallapuram hill near the Mahishamardini cave. It has a facade, *mukha-mandapa* and *ardha-mandapa* like the Kotikal cave. Slim four-sided pillars create space for the two *mandapas*. Its *ardha-mandapa* is about three inches above the *mukha-mandapa*. The facade has two pillars and two pilasters, as does the space separating the two *mandapas*.

"Ramanuja

"One of the most sophisticated and complete cave temples, Ramanuja had three cells. It was excavated in the center of the main Mamallapuram hill, on its eastern scarp. The temple was partially renovated centuries after its construction into a shrine for the Vaishnava scholar, Ramanuja. The later artisans added the six crudely cut, free-standing pillars in front, probably to extend the *mandapa.*

"Koneri

"The Koneri *mandapa,* dedicated to Shiva, has five cells (shrines) attached to its main hall and is named for the Koneri-pallam tank in front. Carved into the western side of the main hill in Mamallapuram, its facade has an entablature. Its cornice has ten *kudus,* with five interconnected *salas* above it. The temple has two rows of four pillars and two pilasters. The front row is considerably simpler than the row near the shrines, which is intricately carved. The pilasters are four-sided and the pillars are cylindrical.

"Krishna

"The Krishna *mandapa* is a sophisticated cave, with large panels depicting the culture of 7th Century Tamil Nadu. The temple is near the *Descent of the Ganges* bas-relief. Its facade consists of four leonine mythical figures *vyala,* holding pillars, and two pilasters. Behind them is another row of pillars. The walls of the pillared hall depict village life woven into the story of Krishna. Krishna holds Goverdhana Mountain, under which are people, cattle and other animals, in one section.

"Atiranachanda

"The 7th Century Atiranachanda cave temple is in the village of Saluvankuppam, north of Mamallapuram. It has a small facade, with two octagonal pillars with square *sadurams* (bases) and two four-sided pilasters. Behind the facade is an *ardha-mandapa* and a small square sanctum. In front of the facade are empty mortise holes, probably later additions to a now-missing *mandapa.*

"Adivaraha

"The Adivaraha cave temple, also known as the Maha Varaha Vishnu temple, is still in use. It is known for sculptures relating the Hindu legends about Varaha (Vaishnavism), Durga (Shaktism), Gangadhara (Shaivism), Harihara (Vaishnavism-Shaivism fusion) and Gajalakshmi (Vaishnavism). The temple is at the northern end of the main Mamallapuram hill, on its western side. Similar to the Varaha *mandapa*, both have been dated to the 7th century Narasimha Varman era. Although it has later inscriptions consecrating the temple, its style suggests that it was built earlier. The famed *avatara* inscription found in this temple, which places a floruit on the Buddha as the ninth avatara of Vishnu, is dated to mid 7th century.

"Mahishasuramardini

"The Mahishasuramardini cave, also known as the Mahishamardini *mandapa*, is found at the southern end of the site (known locally as Yamapuri). Excavated on the eastern scarp of a boulder on the main Mamallapuram hill, above it are the ruins of the Olakkannesvara temple. According to Ramaswami, the temple is unfinished but what has been carved represents the ultimate in Tamil temple rock art. The cave has many panels, and their narrative follows the *Markandeya Purana*.

"Panchapandava mandapam

"Just south of the *Arjuna's Penance* bas-relief is the Panchapandava mandapam, the largest (unfinished) cave temple excavated in Mamallapuram. It has six pillars, one of which has been restored, and two pilasters as its facade. Another row of pillars follows in the *ardhamandapa* and largely unfinished, deep side halls also contain pillars.

"Shore Temple

"The Shore Temple complex is near the Mamallapuram shore, hence its modern name. It consists of a large temple, two smaller temples and many minor shrines, open halls, gateways, and other elements, much of which is buried by sand. The main temple is within a two-tier, compound wall with statues of Shiva's vahana (vehicle), Nandi, surrounding it. It is a stepped pyramidal tower, arranged in five tiers with Shiva iconography. The temple includes a path around its main sanctum and a large barrel-vaulted roof above its doorway. Pilasters on the outer wall divide it into bays. The temple is steeper and taller than the Arjuna and Dharmaraja *rathas*, with a similar design in which the super structure repeats the lower level in a shrinking square form. An octagonal shikhara and kalasa-(pot)-shaped finials cap the tower.

"Olakkanesvara temple

"The Olakkanesvara temple is perched on the rock above the Mahishamardini cave temple. It is also known as the Old Lighthouse because of its conversion by British officials. The temple, built in the early 8th century from gray granite cut into blocks, is credited to King Rajasimha. It is severely damaged, and its superstructure is missing; what remains is a square building with its west entrance flanked by *dvarapalas*. The walls of the temple depict the Ravananugraha legend from the *Ramayana* and a relief of Dakshinamurti (Shiva as a Yoga teacher).

"Mukundanayanar temple

"The Mukundanayanar temple has *ratha*-like architecture. North of the main hill in Mamallapuram, it has been dated to the early 8th century and attributed to King Rajasimha. The temple, with a simple square design, is oriented to the east and its facade is supported by two slender, fluted, round pillars. Its sanctum is surrounded by granite walls, and its outer walls are articulated into plastered columns. Artisans shaped the roof to resemble timber, and the corners have square domed *kutas* (pavilions). The superstructure is tiered into squares, topped with an octagonal dome. The inside of the superstructure is cut to create a *shikhara* above the *garbhagriha*. There is a square panel in the sanctum, but the image is missing.

"Rock reliefs

"Reliefs are carved on rocks or boulders. These include the wall of the Krishna *mandapa*, where a superstructure was added in front of the relief. The best-known rock relief in Mahablipuram is the *Descent of the Ganges* (also known as *Arjuna's Penance* or *Bhagiratha's Penance*), the largest open-air rock relief.

"The *Descent of the Ganges* is considered one of the largest bas-relief works in the world. The relief, consisting of Hindu literature, is carved on two 27-meter-long-(89-foot)-9-meter-high-(30-foot) boulders.

"The beauty of our temples and related structures is there for the world to see. No civilization in the world has come even close to constructing and carving such brilliant, out-of-the-world sculptures anywhere in the world," Madhu proudly stated as he finished his exhaustive talk on the Temples of Mahabalipuram.

Evening was closing in and Madhu decided to go back to his apartment. Another rendezvous was confirmed for the next day as we parted.

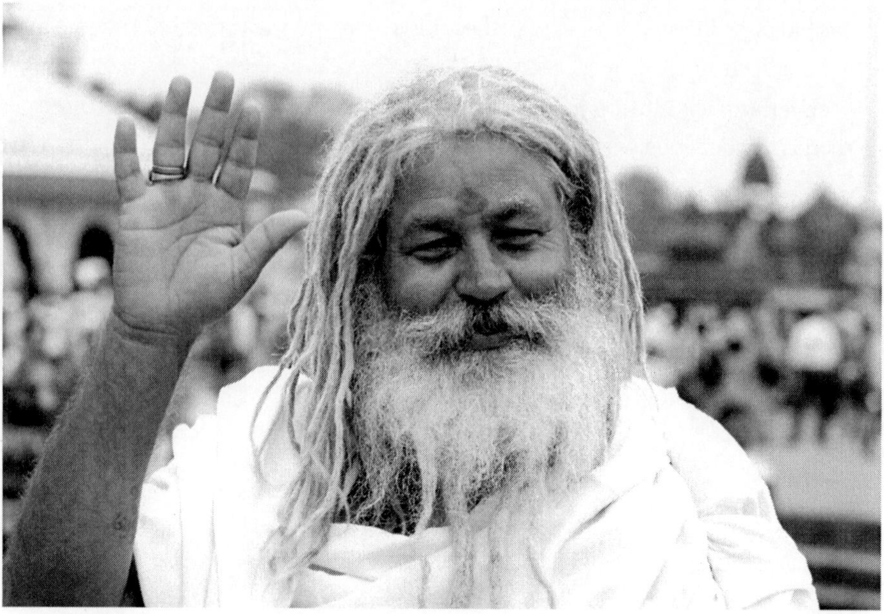

An unidentified Sadhu looks as he participates in the religious event Maha Kumbha Mela in Nashik, India. Credit: ajijchan

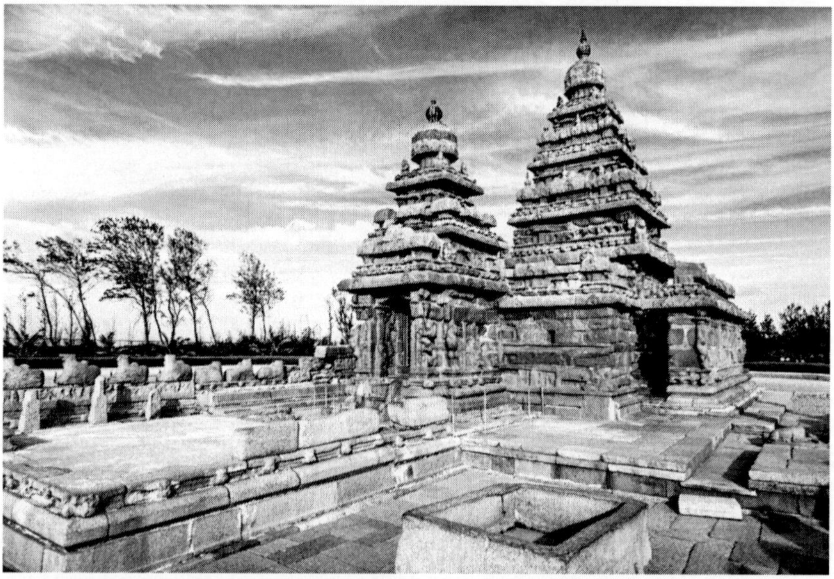

Famous Tamil Nadu landmark- Shore Temple, world heritage site in Mahabalipuram, Tamil Nadu. Credit: f9photos

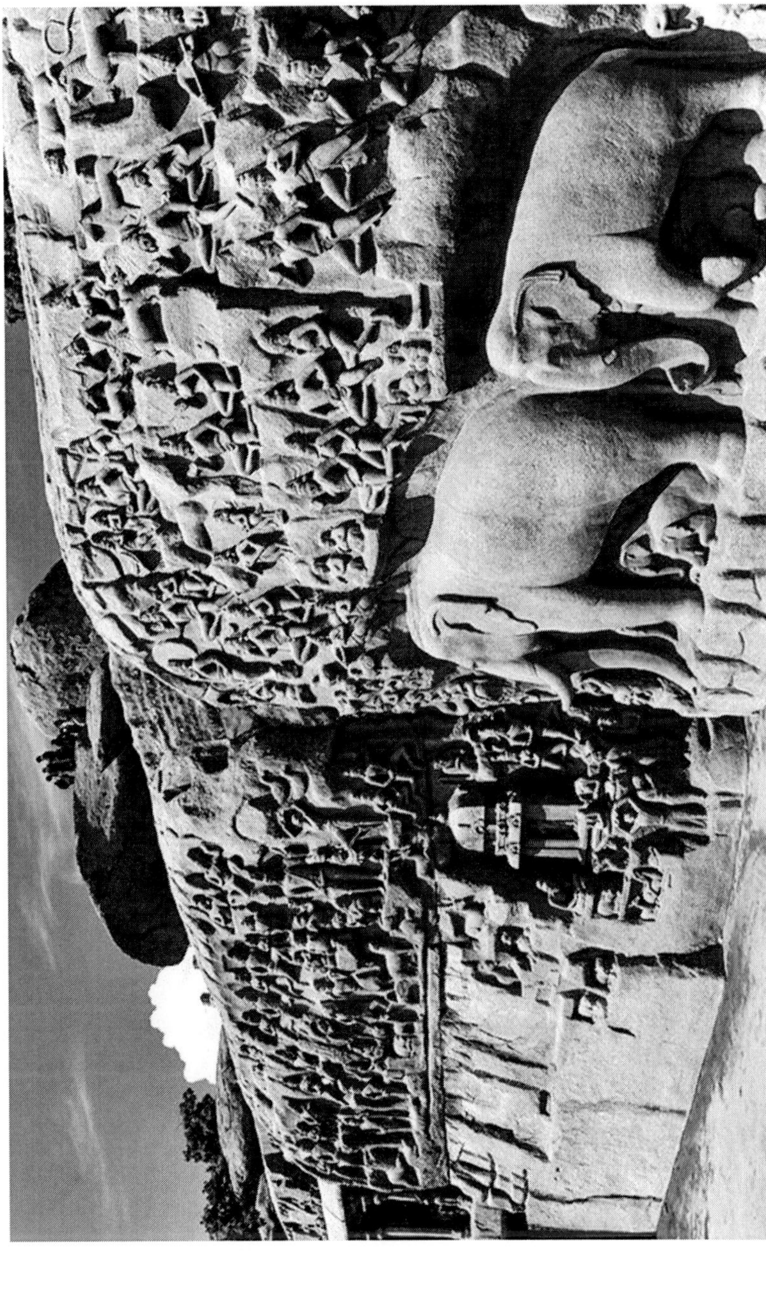

Indian rock cut art of ancient historical animal sculptures at rock cut temples in Tamil Nadu. Credit: Hi

Chapter 8

The Path of Austerities

The first whiff of the approaching winter was evident in the bare branches of trees, and a cool breeze caressing our faces and blowing our scarves. Madhu and I were enjoying a walk in our backyard. Soon it became a little too cold for us and also darkness was descending fast.

We sat on our sofas and were served cups of hot coffee by my wife. A plate of cookies was added for us.

"Shomikda, I have heard so much about our potential and our destination. What are the initial steps?" he asked questioningly.

"Austerities. Austerities can be broadly described as ascetic practices or imposing restrictions on oneself and regulating one's life. In the Bhagavad Gita, Lord Krishna moves to the subject of *yajña* (sacrifice) and explains that based on the modes of nature, sacrifice can manifest into varied forms. He also discusses *tapah* (austerity) and describes the austerities of the speech, body, and mind. Again, based on the modes in which these austerities are performed—goodness, passion, or ignorance, they take different forms. Similarly, *dān* (charity) and its three-fold division based on the modes of nature are explained.

"Austerities performed with body, speech and mind in conjunction with the mode of goodness like meditating for God realization is in the mode of goodness or sattvic. Austerities performed to gain any material possession or position are in the mode of passion, or rajasik. Austerities conducted for using the powers or results to bring harm to someone or for any negative results is in the mode of ignorance or tamasik.

"The sattvic self-discipline of austerities removes physical, emotional and mental impurities. The Bhagavad Gita mentions three categories of austerities:

Physical austerity (of the body), which includes worship, refraining from violence, sexual restraint, honorable behavior and physical purity (e.g., no alcohol or drugs);

Austerity of speech, which includes speaking truthfully and kindly, as well as reciting sacred texts; and

Mental austerity, which includes maintaining calmness, gentleness and self-restraint, as well as meditative practice.

The austerities are interconnected. For example, maintaining physical austerity also develops willpower and mental strength, while the calmness of austerity of the mind promotes austerity of speech.

"Austerity is the tenth and final niyama. Austerity is performing sadhana, penance, tapas and sacrifice. So, we have a four-fold definition of austerity here: sadhana, penance, tapas and sacrifice.

"It sounds like a lot of possibly unpleasant work. I will just watch a game on TV. Why bother with the whole process? What is the benefit?

"Well, it is evolving our consciousness through austerities to help in our spiritual path. Stated differently, it is increasing the speed at which our soul body is maturing. Put in gardening terms, we are fertilizing our soul body. It is going to grow a lot faster. We are fertilizing it. We are giving it what it needs to grow: sadhana, austerities, tapas and sacrifice.

"We are also resolving our karma at a quicker speed, which means it takes fewer lifetimes to go through the process. If we want to hang around a lot, see the mess going on here. But if we want to move on, experience the grandeur of our spiritual being faster, then this is definitely the fertilizer we need. "The theme that goes through all four aspects of austerity is purification. As the intense fire of the furnace refines gold to brilliance, so does the scorching suffering of austerity purify the soul to resplendence.

"So, purification can sometimes cause a sense of suffering. But it is for a good cause. It is getting rid of the impurities. Not just suffering because you are supposed to suffer, it is a reaction to the process of purification.

"The simplest form, of course, is our daily sadhana. Daily sadhana gets us going at a certain rhythm, a certain smoothness in life, a certain rate of moving forward. But that is all based upon maintaining the daily sadhana. If we stop our sadhanas, our life is going to change. It is being supported at that level of sublimity, that level of success, by our sadhana.

"We are also encouraged to go to the temple once a week, at least, and attend festivals. The yearly pilgrimage to a far-off temple is the last part of that.

"Penance, of course, is atoning for misdeeds. It is easy to know if we should do penance because we feel bad about something we did. We cannot get it off our mind. It is just sitting there, nagging us. Wake up in the morning and there it is. Dream about it at night, think about it during the day. The subconscious is telling us, "Hey, there is something down here to be resolved." It keeps throwing it up. So, it is easy to know when penance should be performed and doing so softens the karma, mitigates the karma involved in whatever it is that we have done.

"Simple penances as we know are like prostrations, a hundred and eight prostrations. A little more intense is walking prostrations. We have the ability here to do walking prostrations on the path to Jagannath Puri temple.

"For us grihastas or householders, intense austerities are not practical. We should do each duty in our lives as an act of worship. We should work to offer everything as a prayer and offering to God. His Holy Name should be chanted with every breath. Some things need to be grafted into our lives and in the lives of our children. Prayers in the morning, while bathing, while eating, while going out, during the day, at night before sleeping, prayers and remembrance of the Lord should be a part of routine, not an occasional accident. The parents need to take responsibility from childhood of that practice. It creates children who are more balanced, more loving, honest, and have integrity, more happy, more peaceful, more stoic, and never get into the ordinary folks' banter on unproductive and low-level talks. Creation of a better generation starts from childhood. We need to help them inculcate and exemplify good qualities and attitudes right from childhood, actually from their time they are in the womb.

"I have explained the process of OM Kriya Yoga, in the next few chapters. It lays down the process of Kundalini Yoga as I have learnt and practiced. It is important that we learn and follow some system of authentic sadhana and follow it to the core. That is the secret of success. Sadhana is life. Sadhana should be done all through our lives at every moment. Being in the consciousness is most important, being meditative whenever we can, is also important. Sitting to be meditative is one option. It should be an endeavor all the time.

"You do not need to leave everything and go to the forests, or monastery, or in seclusion. If your mind can be detached, you can be in mental seclusion all the time. And without it, you can be in bondage all the time, even in a monastery or the forests.

"It is my request to the parents of this generation to learn parenting and supporting the growth and development of good children through our time-tested and time-honored systems prescribed in our scriptures. The scriptures in India are based on Dharma or the Cosmic Laws. That is why our civilization is in tune with Nature at every level. Please follow our scriptures and raise good global citizens whom the succeeding generations can look up to."

Madhu seemed to be in a trance while listening to my talk. He stirred as I ended and said, "Shomikda, you seem to have a solution for everything."

I said, "No, I have matured with age and experience and that what gives me the knowledge to say everything. Also, I had the blessing to associate with God-realized saints who move around as ordinary men amongst us but are highly elevated.

"Let me talk about another ancient temple complex in Halebid, where I had visited. [34]Located in Hassan district, the small town of Halebeedu once served as the regal capital of the Hoysala Empire (10th to 14th centuries) and attracts tourists from all parts of the country for its magnificent temples. The prime attractions in Halebeedu are the twin temples of Hoysaleshwara and Kedareshwara. The twin temple complex houses two grand statues of Nandi (bull god), Lord Shiva's vehicle. People can see as many as 108 pillars inside the temple. These pillars resemble each other but feature different design patterns. The temple walls are adorned with intricate carvings of Hindu deities like Lord Brahma, Lord Vishnu and Lord Shiva. They also feature scenes from Hindu epics like the Mahabharata, along with finely carved images of animal figures like elephants and horses. The temple also houses a separate sanctum dedicated to Lord Surya, the Sun God.

"Some of the temples in the Halebid are:

"Hoysaleswara Temple, which is the largest and most elaborate, a twin temple dedicated to Shiva with a major display of reliefs of Shaivism, Vaishnavism, Shaktism and Vedic legends.

"Then there are Jain temples, Halebidu—three large temples in a row,

[34] *Incredibleindia.org.*

close to Hoysaleswara, dedicated to Parshvanatha, Shantinatha and Adinatha of Jainism, major monolith Jina statues and intricately carved Saraswati.

"Kedareshwara Temple, Halebidu, is a three-sanctum temple dedicated to Lord Shiva, also with a galaxy of reliefs of Shaivism, Vaishnavism, Shaktism and Vedic legends.

"Northern group of historic Hindu and Jain temples houses a much simpler architecture and limited artwork but living temples with ruins recovered by local community; these include the Gudlesvara, Virabhadra, Kumbalesvara and Ranganatha temples.

"Nagaresvara and palace archaeological sites have mounds and ruins; excavations of a few mounds have unearthed Hindu and Jain temple structures, idols and scattered parts.

"Hulikere step well is one of the most sophisticated 12th Century step wells in South Karnataka, illustrating the public water infrastructure in erstwhile Hoysala capital.

"Museum is a park and near the Hoysaleswara temple.

"Some other structures are:

"Chennakeshava Temple, Belur—near Halebidu, Belur, was the first capital of the Hoysalas. The Chennakeshava temple is the largest pre-14th Century Kar- nataka tradition Hindu temples complex that has survived into the modern age. "Bucesvara Temple, Koravangala—a twin temple near Hassan city that synthesizes the pre-Hoysala traditions of Hindu architecture, includes artwork from all three major Hindu traditions; about 35 kilometers (22 miles) southeast of Halebidu.

"Nageshvara-Chennakeshava Temple complex, Mosale, is another major temple complex that presents Shaivism and Vaishnavism traditions together, about 20 kilometers (12 miles) northeast of Halebidu.

"Veera Narayana Temple, Belavadi, is a major three-sanctum temples complex, about 25 kilometers from Belur, with beautiful carvings, preserved Vesara superstructure and a galaxy of artwork from all Hindu traditions, about 12 kilometers (7.5 miles) north of Halebidu.

"Lakshminarasimha Temple, Javagal, is a triple-sanctum shrine from the 13th-century, with a galaxy of artwork from all Hindu traditions; a Vesara architecture, where the aedicule on the outer walls shows many major variants of Dravida and Nagara *shikhara* (superstructure) styles; it is about 12 kilometers (7.5 miles) northeast from Halebidu.

"Lakshminarasimha Temple, Haranhalli, and Someshvara Temple, Haranhalli, are sets of Hindu temples from 1234 C.E., with a complex two-story Vesara-architecture, one dedicated to Vishnu avatars and the other to Shiva, but they include major reliefs of Vaishnavism, Shaivism and Shaktism; about 30 kilometers (19 miles) east from Halebidu.

"Ishvara Temple, Arasikere, is a Vesara and Hoysala architecture Hindu temple for Shiva that illustrates the dome-style Hindu architecture for mandapa built about a hundred years before the first invasion of Delhi Sultanate and the start of Deccan version of the Indo-Islamic architecture. It is about 40 kilometers east-northeast of Halebidu.

"Lakshmi Devi Temple, Doddagaddavalli, is one of the earliest Hoysala temples, four sanctums and beautifully carved: about 18 kilometers (11 miles) south of Halebidu.

"Shravanabelagola, Channarayapatna: a major group of many Jain and Hindu monuments; it is about 75 kilometers (47 miles) southeast from Belur on National Highway 75, one of the most important Digambara Jainism pilgrimage sites in South India.

"Nuggehalli group of temples are about 80 kilometers (50 miles) to the east of Halebidu, with the Lakshminarasimha temple featuring an ingenious structure that makes three sanctums appear as one sanctum from outside, which is a Vesara architecture from the 13thcentury. The other major temple in the village, called the Sadasiva Temple, Nuggehalli, is a remarkable Hoysala synthesis of North Indian Nagara architecture with South Indian ideas on architecture."

Madhu was quiet after describing the temple complexes of Halebid, the erstwhile Hoysala capital.

"Shomikda, what treasures we have, especially in the South of India, which are less ravaged by the invaders. Each monument is a world-class display of perfection in sculpture on the hardest rocks. However, in the past seventy years or so, we chose to show the world one monument in India and ignore the actual treasures."

"That is the problem with our freedom. The British continued their rule through proxies," I said, turning slightly political.

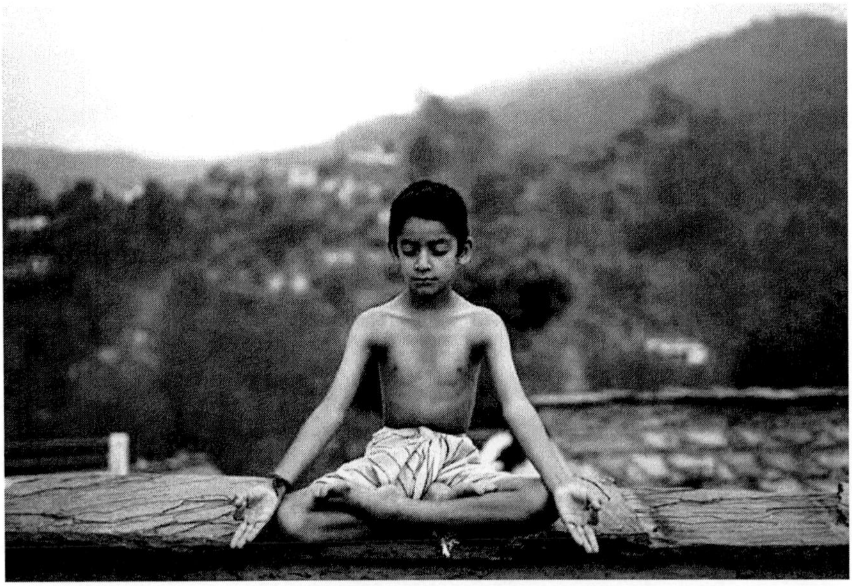

Indian boy doing yoga and meditating, exercising with focus and concentration early morning. Credit: Yogendra Singh

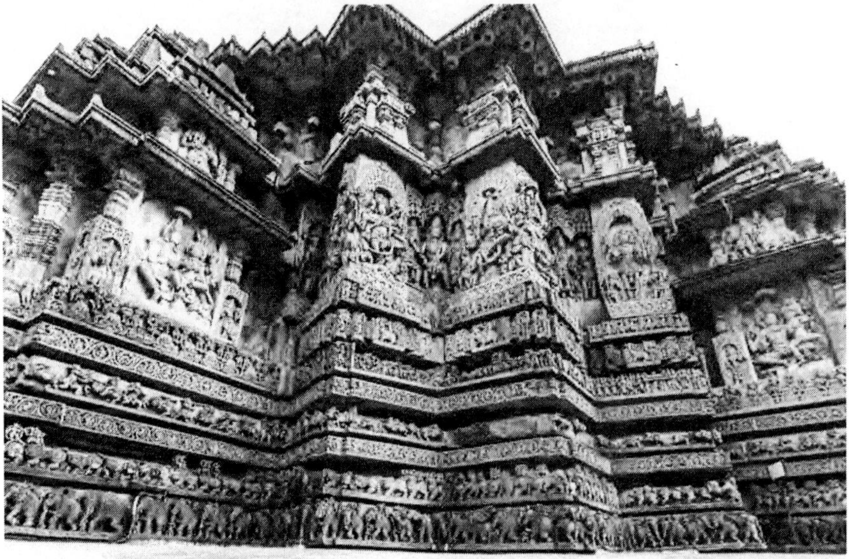

Hoysaleshwara Temple of Lord Shiva. Statues on the Wing of the temple building. Gray and brown stone against light blue sky. Credit: ClaudineVM

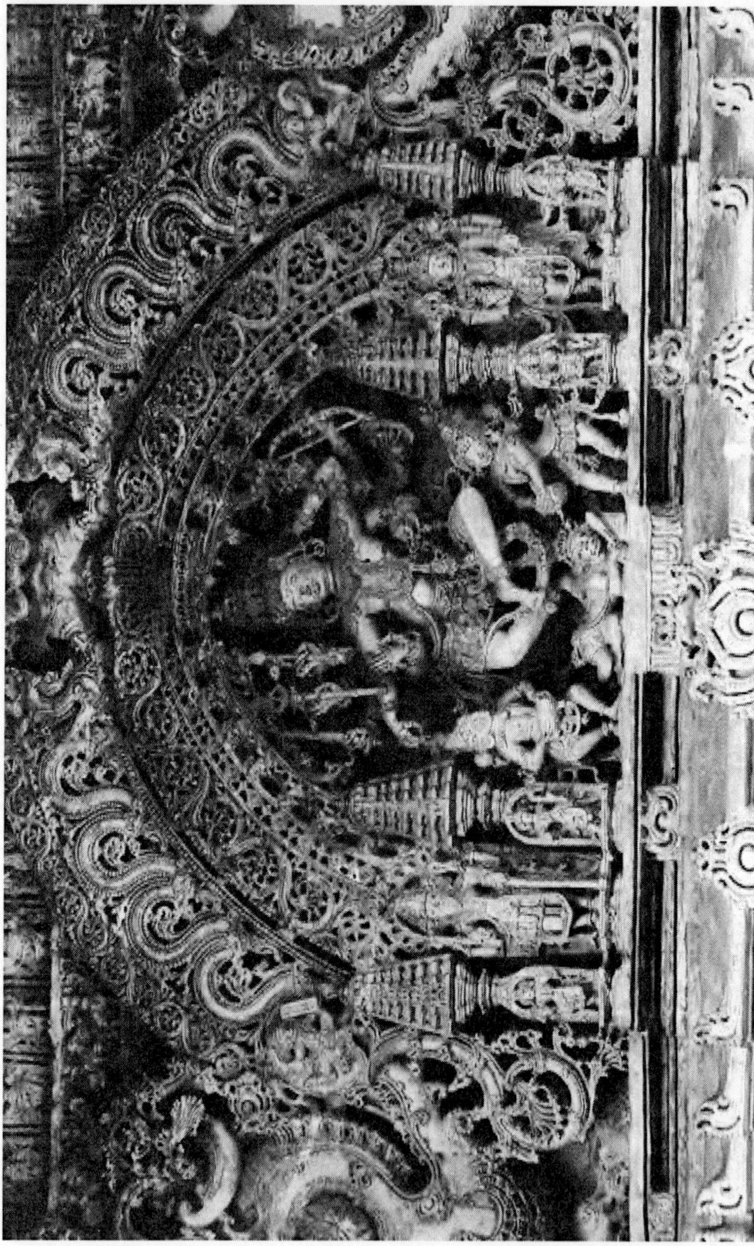

Sculptures on the outer walls of Hoysaleswara Temple at Halebidu, the former capital of the Hoysala.
Credit: Vinayak Jagtap

Chapter 9
Yoga

Madhu and I met again on a holiday celebrating Thanksgiving at our house.

"Shomikda, please talk about Yoga today," Madhu requested me while sipping orange juice on our sofa.

I said, "It is a vast subject. I will try to explain Patanjali's Yoga Sutras in a concise fashion."

Then after another sip of the orange juice, I continued, "To perform the boat posture simply to get a flatter tummy is missing the boat, according to Patanjali.

[35]"Patanjali was the person who codified his thoughts and knowledge of Yoga in *The Yoga Sutra of Patanjali.* In this work, Patanjali compiled 195 sutras, or concise sayings, that are essentially an ethical blueprint for living a moral life and including the science of Yoga into our lives. Although no one is sure of the exact time when Patanjali lived and wrote down his sutras, it is estimated this yogi, who became one of the world's greatest sages, roamed India somewhere between 200 B.C. and 200 A.D.

"In a world where we reduce nearly everything to quick tips and sound bites, Patanjali seems to fit right in with his brief 195 guidelines to enlightenment. But in the case of Patanjali, simplicity is deceptive. In fact, scholars still don't agree on what Patanjali meant in some of his sutras.

"*The Yoga Sutra* is considered the fundamental text on the system of Yoga, and yet you won't find the description of a single posture or asana in it. This

[35] An Autobiography of a Yogi, by Paramahansa Yogananda.

is a guide for living the right life. Essentially, Patanjali says, you can't practice asanas in Yoga class, feel the stretch, and then go home to play cards, cook a meal, abuse your employees, and commit fraud on your taxes. There is more to Yoga than that—Yoga can help you cultivate body, mind, and spiritual awareness.

"The heart of Patanjali's teachings is the eightfold path of Yoga. It is also called the eight limbs of Patanjali, because they interweave like the plants that do the same on a tree in the forest. These aren't directives (although they sometimes sound like them), laws, or hard-and-fast rules. These are Patanjali's recommendations for living a better life through Yoga. Here are the eight limbs of Patanjali.

"Yama "*Yama* is social behavior, how you treat others and the world around you. These are moral principles. Sometimes they are called the 'don'ts' or the 'thou shalt nots.' There are five yamas:

Nonviolence (*ahimsa*). Do no harm to any creature in thought or deed. But you have the right to defend yourself.

Truth and honesty (*satya*). Tell no lies. Cheating in business deals falls into this category.

Nonstealing (*asteya*). Do not steal material objects (a jewel) or intangibles such as the center of attention or your child's chance to learn responsibility or independence by doing something on his own.

Nonlust (*brahmacharya*). Don't worry; this is not a call to celibacy. Many yogis of old were married and had families of their own. The person who practices brahmacharya avoids meaningless sexual encounters and see divinity in all.

Nonpossessiveness (*aparigraha*). Free yourself from greed, hoarding, and collecting. Do you really need more shirts, another car, or to take over the conversation every time you see your friends? Make your life as simple as possible.

"Niyama "*Niyama* is inner discipline and responsibility, how we treat ourselves. These are sometimes called observances, the 'do's,' or the 'thou shalts.' There are five niyamas:

Purity (*shauca*). Purity is achieved through the practice of the five yamas, which help clear away the negative physical and mental states of being. Keep yourself, your clothing, and your surroundings clean. Eat fresh and healthy food. Treat your body like a temple and think of this niyama.

Contentment (*santosha*). Cultivate contentment and tranquility by finding happiness with what you have and who you are. Seek happiness in the moment, take responsibility for where you are, and choose to grow from there.

Austerity (*tapas*). Show discipline in body, speech, and mind. The purpose of developing self-discipline is not to become ascetic, but to control and direct the mind and body for higher spiritual aims or purposes.

Study of the sacred text (*svadhyaya*). Study sacred scriptures, which are whatever books are relevant to you and inspire and teach you. Education changes a person's outlook on life. As Yoga Master B.K.S. Iyengar says, a person starts "to realize that all creation is meant for *bhakti* (adoration) rather than for *bhoga* (enjoyment), that all creation is divine, that there is divinity within oneself and that the energy which moves him is the same that moves the entire universe."

Living with an awareness of the Divine (*ishvara-pranidhana*). Be devoted to God, or whatever you consider divine.

"**Asana** '"The posture of Yoga is steady and easy,' Patanjali says. Patanjali compares this to resting like the cosmic serpent on the waters of infinity. Although Westerners often consider the practice of asana or postures as an exercise regimen or a way to stay fit, Patanjali and other ancient yogis used asana to prepare the body for meditation. To sit for a lengthy time in contemplation required a supple and cooperative body. If you are free of physical distractions—such as your foot going to sleep—and can control the body, you can also control the mind. Patanjali said, "Posture is mastered by freeing the body and mind from tension and restlessness and meditating on the infinite."

"**Pranayama** "*Prana* is the life force or energy that exists everywhere and flows through each of us through the breath. *Pranayama* is the control of breath. The basic movements of pranayama are inhalation, retention of breath, and exhalation. 'The yogi's life is not measured by the number of days but by the number of his breaths,' says Iyengar. 'Therefore, he follows the proper rhythmic patterns of slow, deep breathing.' The practice of pranayama purifies and removes distractions from the mind, making it easier to concentrate and meditate.

"**Pratyahara** "*Pratyahara* is withdrawal of the senses. Pratyahara occurs during meditation, breathing exercises, or the practice of Yoga postures—any time when you are directing your attention inward. Concentration, in the Yoga room or the boardroom, is a battle with distracting senses. When you master pratyahara, you are able to focus because you no longer feel the pain in your stomach or hear the cacophony of sounds from outside or smell the sweetmeats warming up in the microwave.

"**Dharana** "Concentration, or *dharana,* involves teaching the mind to focus on one point or image. 'Concentration is binding thought in one place,' says Patanjali. The goal is to make the mind tranquil—gently pushing away needless thoughts—by fixing your mind on some object such as a candle flame, a point, or a mantra. In dharana, concentration is effortless. You know the mind is concentrating when there is no sense of time passing.

"**Dhyana** "Uninterrupted meditation without an object is called *dhyana.* Concentration (dharana) leads to the state of meditation. The goal of meditation is not unconsciousness or nothingness. It is heightened awareness and oneness with the universe. How do you tell the difference between concentration and meditation? If there is awareness of distraction, you are only concentrating and not meditating. The calm achieved in meditation spills over into all aspects of your life—during a hectic day at work, shopping for groceries, coordinating the Diwali party at your child's school.

"**Samadhi** "The ultimate goal of the eightfold path to Yoga is *samadhi,* or absolute bliss. This is pure contemplation, super-consciousness, in which you and the universe are one. Those who have achieved samadhi are enlightened. Paramahansa Yogananda, author of *An Autobiography of a Yogi,* called it the state of God-Union.

The eight limbs work together: The first five steps—yama, niyama asana, pranayama, and pratyahara—are the preliminaries of Yoga and build the basis for spiritual life. They are concerned with the body and the brain. The last three, which would not be possible without the previous steps, are concerned with reconditioning the mind. They help the yogi to attain enlightenment or the full realization of oneness with Spirit. Enlightenment lasts forever, while a flat tummy can disappear with a week of binging."

As I stopped and took another sip on the orange juice glass, Madhu exclaimed, "Wow. You seem to know so much!"

I said, "Madhu, no use of accolades, which you give so generously. Tell me about the cave temples of Badami. It has the connection with Sage Agastya."

Madhu settled comfortably in his sofa and started, [36]"Badami, formerly known as Vatapi, is a town in the Bagalkot district of Karnataka, India. It was the regal capital of the Badami Chalukyas from 540 to 757 A.D. It is famous for its rock-cut monuments such as the Badami cave temples, as well as the structural temples such as the Bhutanatha temples, Badami Shivalaya and Jambulingesvara Temple. It is located in a ravine at the foot of a rugged, red sandstone outcrop that surrounds Agastya Lake.

"Badami has been selected as one of the heritage cities for HRIDAY—Heritage City Development and Augmentation Yojana scheme of Government of India.

"The Badami region was settled in prehistoric times, as is evidenced by megalithic dolmens.

"In the local tradition, the town of Badami is linked to the Agastya legend of the epics. In the Mahabharata, the asura Vatapi would become a goat, be cooked by his brother Ilvala, and be eaten. Following this, he would recollect in the stomach and tear himself out from the inside of the victim, killing the victim. When the sage Agastya arrives, Ilvala offers the goat to him. However, Agastya, who is known for his enormous powers of ingestion and digestion, kills Vatapi by digesting the meal and giving Vatapi no time to recollect. Agastya thus kills the demons Vatapi and Ilvala. This legend is believed to have played out near Badami, hence the names Vatapi and Agasthya Lake.

"Pulakeshin I, an early ruler of the Chalukyas, is generally regarded as having founded the Badami Chalukya dynasty in 540. An inscription record of this king engraved on a boulder in Badami records the fortification of the hill above 'Vatapi' in 544. Pulakeshin's choice of this location for his capital was likely due to strategic considerations, as Badami is protected on three sides by rugged sandstone cliffs. His son Kirtivarman I and his brother Mangalesha constructed the cave temples located there. The Agastya Lake (formerly Vatapi Lake) is a manmade lake, a water infrastructure project completed in the 7th century, likely as a strategic source of water for the capital and around which many Hindu temples were constructed.

"Badami has eighteen inscriptions, with important historical information. The first Sanskrit inscription in old Kannada script on a hillock dates back to

[36] *IncredibleIndia.org.*

543 C.E., from the period of Pulakeshin I (Vallabheswara); the second is the 578 C.E. cave inscription of Mangalesha in Kannada language and script; and the third is the Kappe Arabhatta records, the earliest available Kannada poetry in *tripadi* (three-line) meter. One inscription near the Bhuthanatha temple also has inscriptions dating back to the 12th century in Jain rock-cut temple dedicated to the Tirtankara Adinatha.

"The Badami cave temples were likely fully painted inside by the late 6th century. Most of these paintings are now lost, except for the mural fragments, bands and faded sections found in Cave 3 (Vaishnava, Hindu) and Cave 4 (Jain). The original murals are most clearly evidenced in Cave 3, where inside the Vishnu temple there are paintings of secular art as well as murals that depict legends of Shiva and Parvati on the ceiling and in parts less exposed to the natural elements. These are among the earliest known paintings of Hindu legends in India that can be dated.

"The façade of the Vishnu temple cave is nearly seventy feet wide, which makes it the largest temple of the lot. There are high relief carvings of Vishnu seated on the coiled serpent Sheshnag, regarded as the most beautiful sculpture of the 16th Century A.D. The cave temple also has exquisite sculptures of Para- sudeva, Bhuvaraha, Harihara, and Narasimha."

Madhu, too, stopped to sip some orange juice from his glass and said, "Shomikda, my sojourn into various parts of India, especially the temples of South India, is the richest experience I have had in my life. The architecture, the sculptures, the energy, all are other worldly. I am a richer person after these experiences," he said with a lot of emotion.

"Yes, indeed, my friend," I ended our discussion for the day.

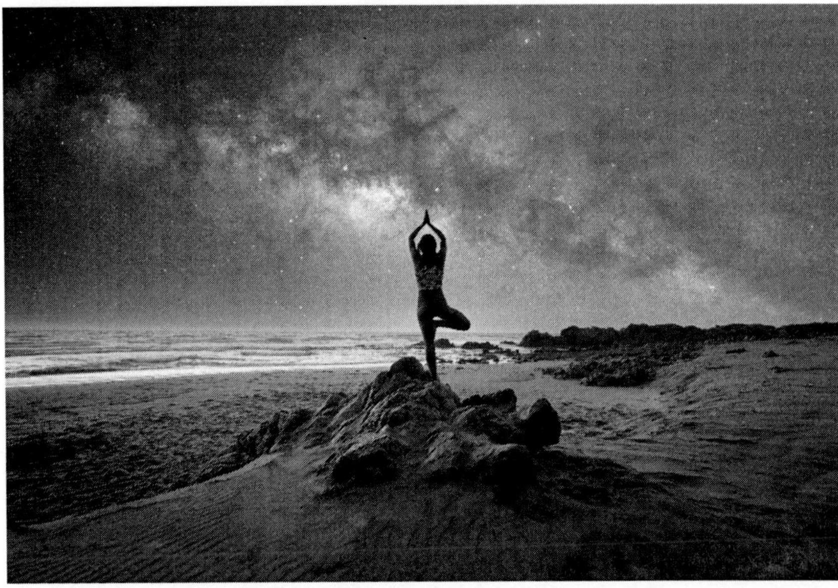

A woman standing in yoga tree position on the beach with the Milky Way background. Credit: Oscar Gutierrez Zozulia

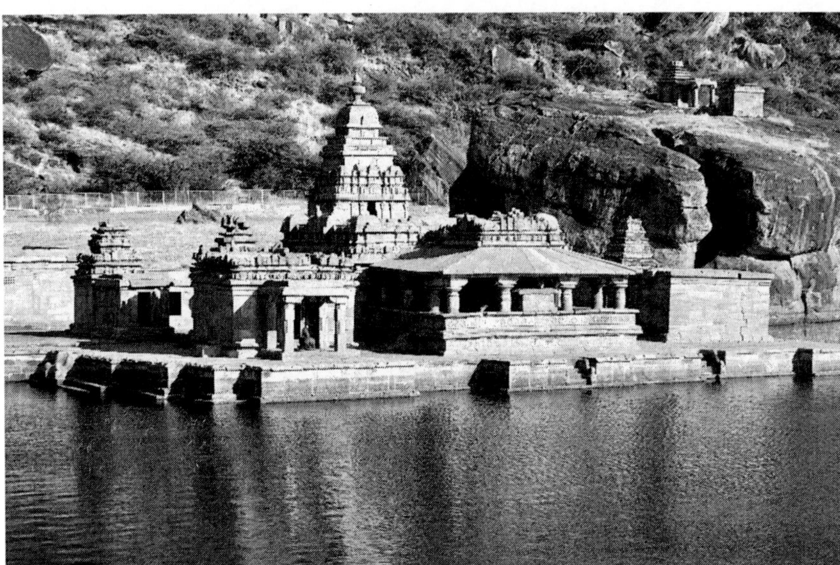

Badami Karnataka India, Bhutanatha temple and Agasthya Tirtha (Lake). Credit: Vinayak Jagtap

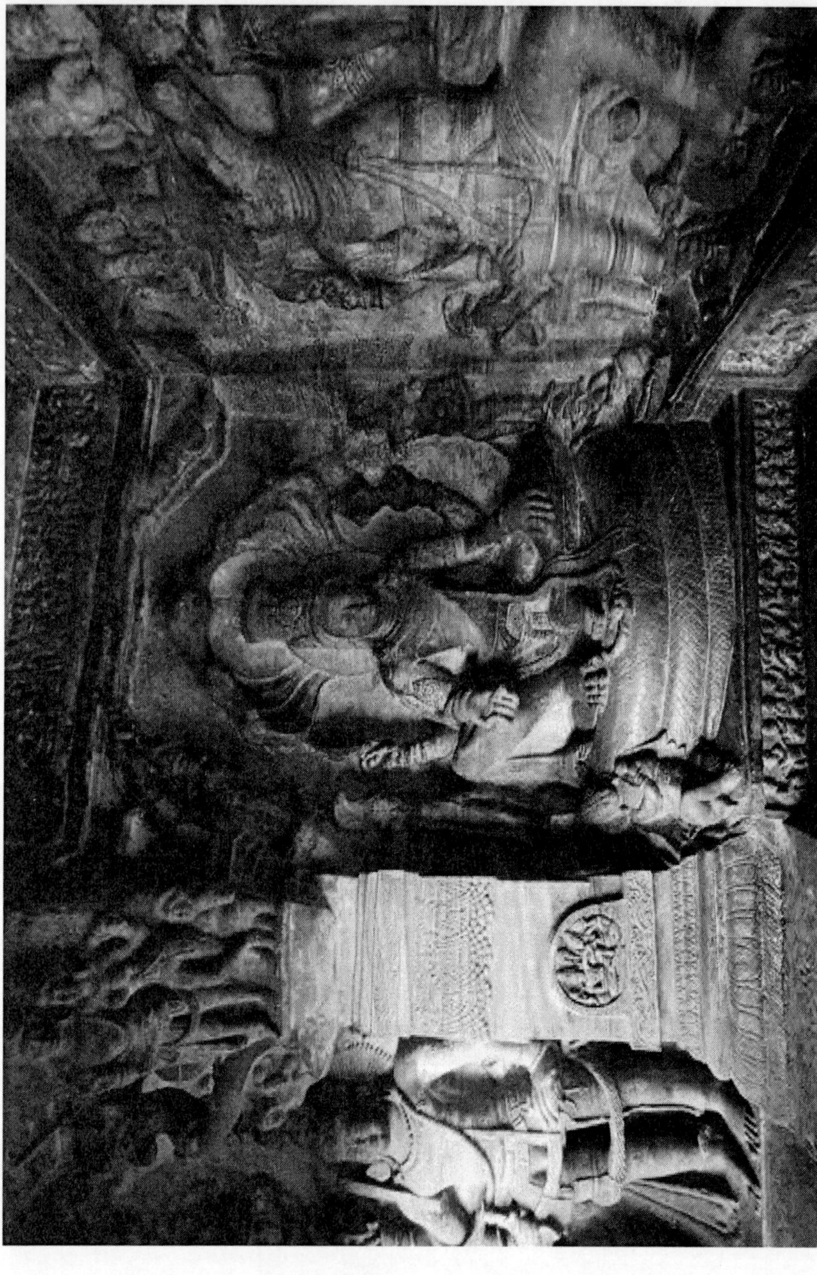

Sculpture of Hindu deities in the Badami Cave Temple.
Credit: ClaudineVM

Chapter 10

OM Kriya Yoga

Madhu came to my house the following day to continue the discussions that we had been having. Along with a cup of coffee and some cookies, our discussion commenced.

I initiated the talk by speaking to him on OM Kriya Yoga, which my revered Guruji, Jagadguru Ramanandacharya Rajivlochanacharya, taught me decades ago.

"I have been practicing Kriya Yoga from childhood days as we were frequented by saints of the highest order. Most of them were men of the world and remained incognito about their spiritual genius. A saint named Satchidananda Sarkar, an author with penname 'Nigurananda,' was a self-realized saint with countless darshans. He initiated us into Kriya Yoga, having received the Shakti Path initiation from Mahavatar Kriya Babaji in the Himalayas. I liked the way he helped us initiate concentration.

"Close your eyes and stare in front of you like you do in the movie theaters. Slowly you will focus only on the 'screen' in front of you, your breath will become shallow and you will lose awareness of the world around you. Focussed concentration commences. That will arouse the Kundalini power and raise your consciousness to higher levels through the Sushumna.

"OM Kriya Yoga taught my revered Guruji, Jagadguru Ramanandacharya Rajivlochanacharya, of Barfani Dham, Indore, the concentration factor but adds some kriyas and asanas to enhance the experience for everyone.

"I met him while working for *News India Times,* the Indian-American newspaper in Manhattan, New York. He was invited by the President of Trinidad and Tobago for a Ramayana event and was invited by the devotees of the USA to come to this country. He was brought to our newspaper office for an interview. The reporter was sick and I took over the responsibility of interviewing him.

"He entered our office as I stood near the door. He was simply light— an effulgence radiated from his being and a spiritual vibration shook me from the innermost core of my existence. He was tall, 6'3" or so, and had a yogic physique. His eyes were like stars and his smile most loving. He was so handsome too.

"I trembled sitting beside him and interviewing him. I came to know that he was the youngest Jagadguru after Adi Shankaracharya, at the age of thirty-six years. He got his direct initiation in OM Kriya Yoga from none other than Mahavatar Kritya Babaji in the Himalayas. He was instructed to spread it globally by Babaji. That is why he was the first Jagadguru to leave the shores of India.

"When I decided to take initiation under his grace, in a few days he touched my head and I could feel energy rushing through my head into my entire being. I was in a trance-like meditative state for the next three-four hours. After that I was a changed person. He gave me the initiated name of 'Yogananda,' a name that I was strangely fascinated by from childhood.

"Before any meditation practice, it is important and useful to practice Pranayama for some time to focus your attention and regulate your breath. It is called Anulom Vilom. Hold the right nostril with your thumb, breathe in through the left. Release through the right nostril, closing the left nostril with the fourth (ring) finger. Inhale from the right nostril and release through the left. Repeat several times slowly, breathing deeply. It clears the lungs of deoxygenated air and fills it with oxygenated air. That fills our cells with energy and you feel rejuvenated and energized. It also removes the toxins in your system.

"Another advance technique of doing pranayama is to count to four while inhaling from the left nostril, holding the breath for sixteen counts and releasing it through the right nostril for eight counts. Focus on each breath and feel the breath consciously. Breathe deep and as long as you can. Then inhale through the right nostril and breathe out through the left. Do this technique for as many minutes as the number of breaths that you take in one minute on any particular day.

"The first step to OM Kriya Yoga is the chanting of OM. 'O' is chanted 25% of the time and 'M' 75% of the time. It is actually AUM, but the 'A' and 'U' combine to become 'O.'

"The kriyas to be followed is to raise the hands above the head straight and chant OM three or eleven times. Imagine that you are getting the power of OM from the environment. Then close your ears with the index fingers and chant OM three or eleven times, imagining that the sound of OM is reverberating inside you. Then you close your eyes with your palms and chant OM three or eleven times. Visualize the radiant OM inside you. Finally place your hands on your knees in [37]Jyana mudra and chant OM three or eleven times. Imagine that OM is in between your eyebrows in the Ajna Chakra and meditate on OM while chanting OM three or eleven times.

"Other than that, there are some kriyas and asanas to arouse the power in the chakras and also to keep the body fit to be able to do sadhana comfortably:

1. **Sukshma Sharir Kriya Sadhana**
   a. Samran Shakti Kriya: Head roll up, down, sideways
   b. Netra Shakti Kriya: Roll eyes up, down, sideways, roll. Same with palms covering your eyes.
   c. Karan Shakti Kriya: Index finger on ears, suck in air, fill mouth, head down, pause, release through nose
   d. Kapol Shakti Kriya: Namaskar pose, close nose with thumb
   e. Giuva/Riva Shakti Kriya: Hang tongue and stretch. Pull your neck and release. Move the head sideways, counterclockwise, up and down.
   f. Kandha Shakti Kriya: Hold breath, lift shoulders, release breath and come back. Keep your fingers on your shoulders and move the hands in a clockwise and counterclockwise direction.
   g. Urja Shakti Bikasak: Extend your fingers, close your fist, pull the energy, and rub over your body.
   h. Bhoja Palli Shakti Kriya: Palms up and down from the wrist after extension. Extend your hands and life up and down your palms. Close the fists and move them in a clockwise and counter-clockwise direction. Lift up your hand with a fist and move the hands

[37] "Jyana Mudra "is when the palms are facing upward and the index finger touches the thumb in each hand.

around your head in a circular motion. Bring your fists near the chest and forcefully breathe out and forcibly push the hands in front.

i. Bacchastal Shakti Kriya: Fill your lungs with air, hands out in front. Then breathe out, extend your arms to the sides and lift yourself on your toes. Repeat with hands going up above our heads and bring them down while breathing out.
j. Kati Shakti Kriya: Hands stretched in front, turn to the right and then left, breathing out. Then put your hands on your hips and move in a circular motion clockwise and counterclockwise directions.
k. Udar Shakti Kriya: Press stomach repeatedly. Take out the air, hold breath and press the stomach repeatedly. Then fill with air and then repeat.
l. Kundalini Shakti Kriya: Pull rectum from inside and release repeatedly. Then hit your back with your legs.
m. Jhanu Shakti Kriya: Bring the legs together and hold the knees and move them around in a clockwise and counterclockwise movement.
n. Panja Shakti Kriya: Legs together, bring right foot and move it up, down and in a circular movement clockwise and counter clockwise. Repeat on the left leg.
o. Prandour: Lift your right leg at the back and move your left fist forward. Your right fist should be near your chest. Repeat the left leg and the right hand. Increase your speed. Breathe out strong.
p. Sabasana: Total relaxation in a corpse pose.

2. Chakra Kriya Asanas:

a. *Halasana*

1. Sit at the front end of your mat and lie back over the blankets so they support your torso. Adjust your position so that the tops of your shoulders are about an inch over the edge and the back, your head rests on the floor. Lie face up so that the front of your neck is long and there's space between the back of your neck and the floor.
2. Bring your knees toward your chest, then straighten your legs toward the ceiling.

3. Using the strength of your abs—and supporting yourself with both hands at your lower or mid-back—lift your hips off the floor and roll up until you are supported by your shoulders. Stack your hips above your shoulders.
4. Slowly lower your legs backward over your head until your toes reach the ground behind you. Rest your toes on the ground, feet flexed.
5. Release your hands and place your arms on the floor, palms down or with hands clasped. Press down with your outer upper arms and shoulders to create more lift along the spine.
6. Hold for five breaths or more.
7. To exit, unclasp your hands, press your arms and hands into the mat, and slowly roll down one vertebrae at a time.
8. Take a few moments to allow the back to settle back into its normal curves.

b. *Sarvangasana*

1. Exhaling, raise high the legs together enough to make a right angle with the body. Keep the knees straight and the body above the hip-joint on the ground undisturbed.
2. At this stage, still exhaling, raise the arms and hold the waist and push the body up as far as possible. Put all the body-weight on the arms and rest on the elbows, with the legs thrown upwards.
3. When this position is firmly secured, by careful manipulation, make an attempt to shift the hands slowly toward the waist, with the fingers extended to the back of the hipbones and the thumbs pressed lightly on both sides of the navel.
4. Set the chin in the jugular notch and place the full weight upon the shoulders, the neck and the back of the head (final position). Complete the above steps in four seconds, while exhaling.
5. Maintain this pose as long as convenient, but not longer than two minutes, breathe normally slow, rhythmic and natural.

6. Return to starting position: Slowly bend the knees and then gently lower the hips toward the mat, supported by the hands in four seconds, while inhaling.
7. Release the hands from the back and assume the starting position.
8. Take a few deep breaths and then rest a while, breathe normally.

c. *Sarpasana or Bhujangasana*

1. Lie flat on the stomach with the legs straight and the feet together.
2. Place your hands by the side of your chest. Inhale deeply and slowly.
3. Using the lower-back muscles, raise the chest as far as possible from the floor. Place the hands on the floor and raise the torso as high as possible, pushing from the back.
4. Raise the body as high as possible without straining.
5. Retaining breath, squeeze the shoulder blades together and look forward.
6. Hold for as long as is comfortable.
7. Exhaling, slowly return to the starting position and relax the whole body. Release the hands and relax the arms by the sides of the body. Turn the head to one side.
8. This is one round. Perform up to five rounds.

d. *Dhanurasana*

1. Begin on your belly with your legs hip-distance apart and your palms on the mat beside your lower ribs.
2. Extend your feet straight back and press down with the tops of all ten toenails to activate your quadriceps.
3. Rotate your inner thighs toward the ceiling (to broaden your lower back) and firm your outer ankles into your midline (to prevent your feet from turning inward).
4. Keep your hands on the mat as you lift your head and chest a few inches off the mat and keep a slight tuck of your chin. Roll your shoulders back and up.

5. Bend your knees and reach back with your hands to clasp the outside of your ankles. (Be certain to reach back with both hands at the same time.) This hand position puts your shoulders in internal rotation, so roll your shoulders back and up again.
6. Press your thighs into the mat.
7. Keep your feet flexed and your outer ankles from bowing out. Press the bottoms of your feet up toward the ceiling to energize your legs.
8. Keep your thighs on the mat as you push your shins toward the wall in back of you as you lift and open your chest. Roll your shoulders back again to reinforce the external rotation.
9. Lift your thighs off the mat. Begin with your inner thighs.
10. Relax your glutes.
11. Continue to press your shins back and away from your hands as you reach your sternum forward and up, balancing on your navel.
12. Lift your gaze slightly so the curve of your neck is a continuation of the curve of your upper back.
13. Hold for five to ten breaths. To ease out of the pose, bend your knees and lower your legs to the floor. Then release your grip.

e. *Supta Matsyendraasana*

1. Lying on your back, bring your arms out to the sides with the palms facing down in a T position. Bend the right knee and place the right foot on the left knee.
2. Exhale drop the right knee over to the left side of your body, twisting the spine and low back. Look at the right fingertips.
3. Keep the shoulders flat to the floor, close the eyes, and relax into the posture. Let gravity pull the knee down, so you do not have to use any effort in this posture.
4. Breathe and hold for six to ten breaths.
5. To release: Inhale and roll the hips back to the floor, and exhale the leg back down to the floor.
6. Repeat on other side.

f. *Bajrasana*

1. Start by kneeling on the floor. Consider using a Yoga mat for comfort.
2. Pull your knees and ankles together and point your feet in line with your legs. The bottoms of your feet should face upward with your big toes touching.
3. Exhale as you sit back on your legs. Your buttocks will rest on your heels and your thighs will rest on your calves.
4. Put your hands on your thighs and adjust your pelvis slightly backward and forward until you're comfortable.
5. Breathe in and out slowly as you position yourself to sit up straight by straightening your spine. Use your head to pull your body upward and press your tailbone toward the floor.
6. Straighten your head to gaze forward with your chin parallel to the floor. Position your hands palms down on your thighs with your arms relaxed.

g. *Mandukasana*:

1. Fists on the navel, head on the floor or knees.
2. Comfortably sit in Vajrasana (thunderbolt pose).
3. Close the fists of both hands.
4. While clenching the fists, press your thumb inside with the fingers.
5. While pressing the navel with both of your fists, exhale and bend forward.
6. Hold the breath when you are in the position of bent forward and keep looking straight.
7. Stay in this position for some time (hold the position as much as you can), inhale, and come back to the starting position (Vajrasana).
8. Repeat this three to four times.

h. *Paschimottanasana*

1. Begin seated with your legs straight in front of you. Flex your feet and press your heels away from you.

2. Inhale and sit tall. Exhale and hinge at your hips to lean forward. Lengthen your spine rather than around your back.
3. Walk your hands as far forward as your back and hamstrings allow you to comfortably stretch. If you can reach your feet, loosely rest your hands on the outer edges. Keep your feet flexed with your knees and toes pointing toward the ceiling.
4. With each inhalation, lift and lengthen your chest slightly; with each exhalation, release a little more fully into the forward bend. If your hands are resting on your feet, let your elbows bend out to the sides.
5. Stay in the pose for one to three minutes. To come out, release your feet as you slowly come back to sitting on an inhalation.

i. *Ustrasana, or Camel pose*

1. Come to your knees, with your legs hip-width apart. Keep your hips over your knees and squeeze your thighs toward each other.
2. Inhale, engage your lower belly, and reach your tailbone toward your knees, creating space between your lower vertebrae.
3. On another inhalation, lift your sternum and draw your elbows back, toward each other behind you. Allow your ribcage to expand.
4. Keep your chest raised, your core engaged, your spine long, your chin tucked and your shoulders back as you drop your hands toward your heels.
5. Press the heels of your hands into the heels of your feet, draping the fingers over the soles. Keep lifting through your sternum. (If you don't have the spinal flexibility for full Ustrasana, avoid reaching for your feet; instead, use blocks placed on the outside of each ankle or keep your hands on your hips with your thumbs on your sacrum.)
6. Now lift your shoulders to allow the trapezius muscles between the shoulder blades to rise up and cushion your cervi cal spine. Gently allow the head and neck to extend backward. Gaze at the tip of your nose.

7. Stay in this pose for thirty to sixty seconds. To exit, bring your chin to your chest and your hands to your hips with your thumbs on your sacrum. Engage your lower belly and use your hands to support your lower back as you come slowly back up to your knees.

j. *Kurmasana*:

1. Sit on knees, fists in naval area, bend forward.
2. Sit in Dandasana with your legs straight in front of you and your hands on the floor alongside your hips. Press your thighs into the floor, flex your feet, and lift your chest. Bring your legs to the edges of the mat, with your knees as wide as your shoulders. Take a few breaths here.
3. Bend your knees, and keeping your feet flexed, bring them closer to your hips. Extend your chest and arms forward and down between your legs.
4. Bend your legs even more, so that you can put your shoulders one by one under your knees. (If this is too difficult, continue to work on forward bends.) Once there, stretch your arms out to the sides. Roll your thighs inward and extend your inner heels, without creating tension in the feet. Spread the front of your chest and collarbone forward and down with the help of the pressure of your thighs on the shoulders or upper arms. Push your inner heels down and forward to stretch and straighten your legs. Your inner thighs should remain in contact with your side ribs.
5. Inhale to continue to stretch your arms and chest out to your sides. Exhale to extend your spine farther forward. Do not force your legs; instead relax and exhale to release as far as you can into the pose. If you feel pain under your knees, take your arms slightly forward. Stay for a few breaths, then slowly come out of the pose. Repeat a few times.

k. *Padmasana*:

1. Sitting cross-legged on the floor (Sukhasana), one foot is placed on top of the opposite thigh with its sole facing upward and heel close to the abdomen. The other foot is then placed on the opposite thigh as symmetrically as possible.

l. *Yogamudra:*

1. Sit in easy pose (*sukhasana*), lotus (*padmasana*) or half-lotus.
2. Bring the hands behind your back.
3. Place the right hand in *adi mudra* position, where the thumb turns across the center of the palm, the tip of the thumb rests at the base of the pinky finger, and all four fingers bend to form a fist that covers the thumb.
4. With the left hand, loosely grasp the right wrist.
5. Allow both hands to rest on the lower back.
6. Bend forward as far as you can, resting your forehead comfortably on the floor, a pillow or a block if possible.
7. Feel the stretch in the lower-back muscles.
8. Slowly bring your body out of the posture, one vertebra at a time, head and neck coming up last. Release the hands once your spine is erect again.

m. *Sukhanana*:

1. Same as Padmasana. Only one leg is placed on the other thigh if not just cross-legged.

n. *Hasanana*:

1. Lift your hands above your head, get on top of your toes and laugh your heart out. Repeat.

o. *Sabasana*:

1. Relax in the corpse pose.
2. Sit on the floor with your knees bent, feet on the floor. Lean back onto your forearms.
3. As you inhale, slowly extend your legs with your feet apart and toes turned out equally.
4. Narrow the front of your pelvis and soften (but don't flatten) your lower back. Lift your pelvis off the floor, slightly tuck your tailbone. (You may use your hand to sweep your buttocks away from your lower back.) Lower your pelvis.
5. With your hands, lift the base of your skull away from the back of your neck, creating length. If it's more comfortable, support your head and neck with a folded blanket. Make sure your shoulders are down and away from your ears.

6. Reach your arms toward the ceiling, perpendicular to the floor. Rock slightly from side to side and broaden the back ribs and the shoulder blades away from the spine. Then release your arms to the floor, angled evenly away from the sides of the body.
7. Turn your arms outward and extend them toward the bottom of the mat. Rest the backs of your hands on the floor. Make sure your shoulder blades rest evenly on the floor.
8. Soften your mouth and tongue, and the skin around your nose, ears, and forehead. Let your eyes sink to the back of the head, then turn them downward to gaze at your heart.
9. Stay in this pose for at least five minutes.
10. To exit, exhale and gentle roll onto one side. Take two or three breaths. With another exhale, press your hands against the floor and lift your torso, bringing your head slowly after.

p. **Astral Travel**:

1. While in Sabasana, notice your body parts and then let the subtle body (mentally initially) come out and travel around the world, the Himalayas, the Kailash Mountain, get Lord Shiva's blessings. Hear continuous OM chanting and reach the sun to get full energy.

q. **Shat Chakra Kriya or Kundalini Shakti Kriya**

1. Inhale strong and pull rectum simultaneously (Muladhara chakra). Hands straight up in the air.
2. Inhale strong and pull genitals simultaneously (Swadhisthana chakra). Hands floating on the side facing up, shoulder-high.
3. Inhale strong and pull stomach simultaneously (Manipura chakra). Palms holding knees.
4. Inhale strong and pull chest simultaneously (Anahata chakra). Thumb and forefinger of each hand one on top of each other, facing each other in front of the chest.
5. Inhale strong and pull throat simultaneously (Visuddhi chakra). Palms on each other, resting on the folded feet.
6. Inhale strong and pull third eye simultaneously (Ajna chakra). Forefinger and thumb touching each other facing up, hands resting on the knees.

7. Inhale strong and pull middle of the head simultaneously (Sahasrara chakra). Hands above the head in pranayama posture.
8. Do Pranayama as described above with Anulom Vilom for some time to increase concentration and focus. Hold the right nostril with your thumb, breathe in through the left. Release through the right nostril, closing the left nostril with the ring (fourth) finger. Inhale from the right nostril and release through the left. Repeat several times slowly, breathing deeply.
9. Om Nada chant: Chant OM with hands above head (three times), with ears blocked with forefingers (three times), with eyes closed and palms on the eyes (three times), with Om Kriya Mudra (palms on the knees with the thumb and forefinger touching, facing upwards) (three times). Focus on the Ajna Chakra and visualize light of OM. Take the light of OM to all parts of the body and cleanse them. Immerse in mental OM chant.
10. Guru Dhyana: Seek blessings from your guru if you have one.
11. Guru Mantra: Chant the mantra given by your guru.
12. Dhyana Samadhi: Go deep into meditation.

"These kriyas and asanas help release the toxins in the body, promote good health, release energy, help in becoming meditative and uplift our consciousness to the higher level.

"This is OM Kriya Yoga in short. Anyone who can follow it can become uplifted. The divine energy is all within us. We just have to arouse the infinite energy. If you cannot follow the entire exercises and kriyas, do what you can, especially meditation and energizing the chakras."

I sat back relaxed as Madhu continued to look up in the ceiling in a deeply meditative state. Finally, he got his consciousness back to the earthly plane and he said, "Shomikda, can we practice this invaluable Om Kriya Yoga system?"

I nodded and said, "Of course, it is for everyone who wants to do it irrespective of anything."

"Madhu, tell me about Hampi, another great place for wondrous architecture and temple carvings that you had visited," I requested Madhu.

Madhu started, [38]"Hampi is situated on the banks of the Tungabhadra River in the eastern part of Central Karnataka, near the state border with Andhra Pradesh.

"Hampi is located in hilly terrain formed by granite boulders. The Hampi monuments, comprising the UNESCO world heritage site, are a subset of the wider-spread Vijayanagara ruins. Almost all of the monuments were built between 1336 and 1570 C.E. during the Vijayanagara rule.

"Virupaksha Temple

"The Virupaksha temple is the oldest temple, the main destination for pilgrims and tourists, and remains an active Hindu worship site. Parts of the Shiva, Pampa and Durga temples existed in the 11thcentury; it was extended during the Vijayanagara era. The temple is a collection of smaller temples, a regularly repainted, 160-foot-high gopuram, and is a Hindu monastery dedicated to Vidyaranya of Advaita Vedanta tradition, a water tank (*Manmatha*), a community kitchen, other monuments and a 2,460-foot-earlier-ruined stone market with a monolithic Nandi shrine on the east end.

"The sanctum of the temple has a *mukha-linga;* a Shiva linga with a face embossed with brass. The Virupaksha temple also has smaller shrines for two aspects of Parvati-Pampa and Bhuvaneshwari to the north of the main sanctum. Bhuvaneshwari shrine is of Chalukyan architecture and it uses granite instead of pot stone. The compound has a northern gopura, smaller than the eastern gopura, that opens to the Manmatha tank and a pathway to the river with stone reliefs related to the *Ramayana*. To the west of this tank are shrines of Durga and Vishnu.

"Krishna Temple

"The Krishna temple, also called Balakrishna temple, on the other side of Hemakuta Hill, is about 1 kilometer (0.62 mile) south of Virupaksha temple. It is dated to 1515 C.E.; this part of the Hampi complex is called Krishnapura in inscriptions.

"The temple opens to the east; it has a gateway with reliefs of all ten avatars of Vishnu, starting with Matsya at the bottom. Inside is the ruined temple for Krishna and small ruined shrines for goddesses.

---

[38] *Incredibleindia.org.*

"Achyutaraya Temple

"The Achyutaraya temple, also called the Tiruvengalanatha temple, is about 1 kilometer (0.62 mile) east of Virupaksha temple and a part of its sacred center is close to the Tungabhadra River. It is referred to be in Achyutapura in inscriptions and is dated to 1534 C.E. It is one of the four largest complexes in Hampi. The temple is unusual because it faces north. It is dedicated to Lord Vishnu.

"Vitthala Temple

"The Vitthala temple and market complex is over 3 kilometers (1.9 miles) northeast of the Virupaksha temple, near the banks of the Tungabhadra River. It is the most exquisitely artistic and sophisticated Hindu temple in Hampi, and is part of the sacred center of Vijayanagara. It is unclear when the temple complex was built, and who built it; most scholars date it to a period of construction in the early to mid 16th Century.

"The Hemakuta Hill

"The Hemakuta Hill lies between the Virupaksha temple complex to the north and the Krishna temple to the south. It is a collection of moderately sized monuments that are the best-preserved examples of pre-Vijayanagara and early-Vijayanagara temples and construction. The site has several important inscriptions, is easily accessible and provides views of some parts of Hampi and the fertile agricultural valley that separates the sacred center from the urban core with its royal center.

"The Hazara Rama Temple

"The Hazara Rama temple, referred to as the Ramachandra temple in inscriptions, occupied the western part of the urban core in the royal center section of Hampi. This temple was dedicated to Lord Rama of the *Ramayana* fame, and an avatar of Lord Vishnu.

"Kodandarama Temple

"The Kodandarama temple complex lies near the Tungabhadra River, and is north of Achyutaraya temple. The temple overlooks Chakratirtha, where the

Tungabhadra turns northwards toward the north of India. The riverbanks, considered holy, accommodate a Vijayanagara-era ghat and mandapa facilities for bathing. In front of the temple is a *dipa stambha* (lighting pillar) under a Peepal tree, and inside is a sanctum dedicated to Rama, Sita, Lakshmana and Hanuman.

"Pattabhirama Temple

"The Pattabhirama temple complex is in the southern suburban center outside the sacred center and the urban core, about 500 meters (1650 feet) from the ASI Hampi museum. It was at the nucleus of economic and cultural activity of this suburb, now located northeast of Kamalapura. The complex, also known as Varadevi Ammana Pattana, was likely built in the early 16th century and dedicated to Lord Rama.

"Mahanavami platform

"The Mahanavami platform, also called the 'Great Platform, ''Audience Hall, 'Dasara' or 'Mahanavami Dibba' monument, is within a 7.5-hectare (19-acre) enclosure at one of the highest points inside the royal center (urban core). It has ceremonial structures. It is mentioned in the memoirs of foreigners who visited Vijayanagara, some calling it the 'House of Victory.' The largest monument in this complex has three ascending square stages leading to a large square platform that likely had a wooden mandapa above it. This was burnt down during the destruction of Hampi.

"Square Water Pavilion

"The Square Water Pavilion, also called the Queen's Bath, is in the southeast of the royal center. It has a pavilion, a water basin and a method of moving fresh water to it and taking away wash water and overflows. The basin is enclosed within an ornate, pillared, vaulted bay. Nearby are the ruins of the aqueduct. The modern name of this building, the Queen's Bath, is probably a misnomer because this was a public bath for men and travelers. It is an amazing example of advanced engineering in the past."

Madhu stopped and had a few sips of a hot coffee. After a few pleasantries, he prepared to go with a promise to meet next time soon.

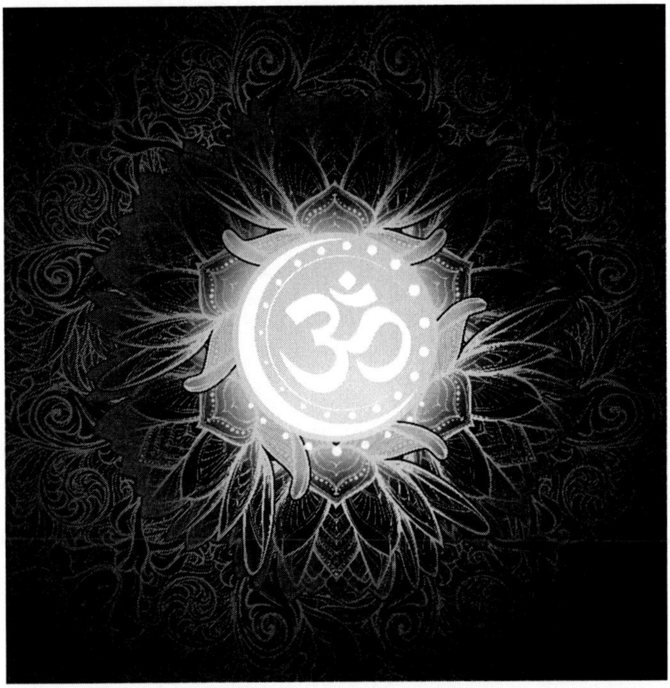

The Primordial Sound of OM in material form. Credit: Anton Tokarev

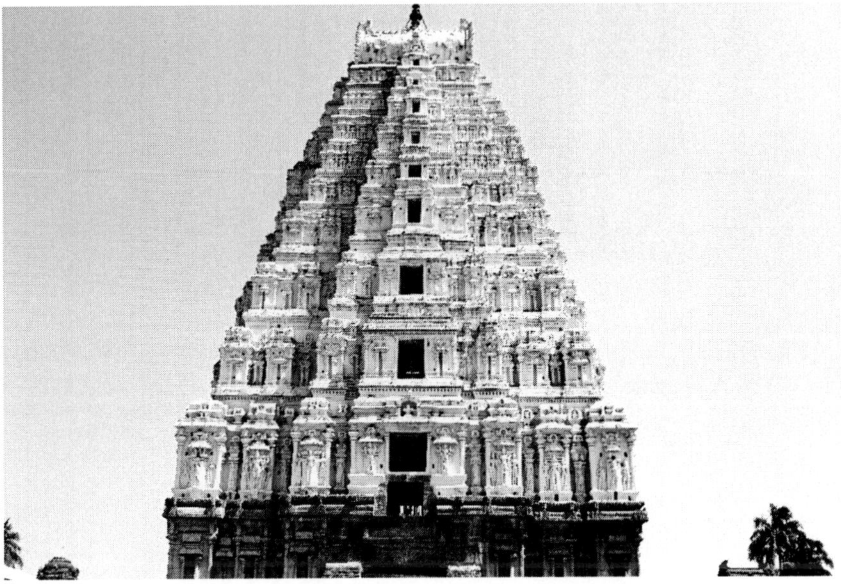

The prominent Virupaksha Temple of Hampi. Credit: Surajit Das

Chapter 11

Mahavatar Kriya Babaji and Jagadguru Ramanandacharya Rajivlochanacharya

Madhu met me the following weekend and we sat on our sofas with our cups of coffee and cookies.

"Shomikda, please tell me something about your revered Guruji. I am so blessed to know the OM Kriya Yoga system from you," he finally said.

"I will definitely talk about my revered Guruji but first you need to know about his Guruji, my Adi-Guruji, Mahavatar Kriya Babaji," I said.

"The Emergence of a Mahavatar[39]

"Though known secretly by Kriya Yogis for centuries, details of the life and birth of the deathless Mahavatar Babaji were not made public until the late 1940s, when the saintly Swami Yogananda Paramahansa was permitted to release a few details of Babaji's incredible incarnation. Later, the great saint included a chapter about Babaji in his magnus opus, *Autobiography of a Yogi.*

In 1952, the celebrated and eternally youthful avatar revealed his birth details to two of his very close disciples. One had authored several books on Kriya Yoga, V.T. Neelakantan. The other was the Tamil Pranayam Siddha, Yogiar S.A.A. Ramaiah.

"Babaji's Birthplace and the Temple upon Which It Sits

"The great master had not revealed any details of his birth prior to the 1950s.In the last few decades, Mahavatar Babaji has become a worldwide phe-

---

[39] Ref: *https://www.yoginiashram.com/babaji/.*

nomenon, particularly among mystics, yogis and tantrics. He works at all levels and has integrated into the consciousness of awakened souls everywhere. He was born in Swethanathapuram, an ancient seaport near Chidambaram, India, on 30 November, 203 A.D. The town is now known as Parangipettai. In the early 1950s, Babaji led Neelakantan and Yogiar to the sacred site at the very beginning of Yogiar's decades-long spiritual mission.

"In 1971, the plot of land where Babaji was born was filled with thorns and rocks, but it was a place of great peace, power and bliss. There were no shade trees and the summer sun of South India was scorching hot.

"A granite temple dedicated to Babaji on the holy site was constructed. The rough granite slabs were quarried near Kanadukathan and moved by bullock cart to the carving location. The carvings and reliefs were performed in the town of Karakudi in the ancient tradition. When the carved blocks and images were complete, and the temple was ready to assemble, all were transported by trucks to Babaji's birthplace. For the next two months of construction, monsoon season peaked and it rained constantly as the deadline approached for dedicating the temple, which had been determined astrologically far in advance. The workers were courageously moving the massive stone blocks with levers as they sloshed through mud and rain chanting the names of God to maintain the rhythm of the work and keep their energy high.

"When the construction was complete, even as the rain continued Brahmin priests placed the astabandha (a special kind of cement) to secure Babaji's moorthi to his pedestal.

"A Blessing from Babaji at the Dedication Ceremony

"Miraculously, as the Mahakumbh Abeshak (the first ceremonial bath) at the sacred hour started, the rains stopped for the very first time in many weeks. The clouds parted and a beam of light descended directly on the temple itself. The light beam remained on the temple until the puja was complete. One single beam of light maintained its position on the temple throughout the puja, while no other light in any direction could be seen.

"Yantras and other secret things of which I cannot speak were placed strategically and in a safe hidden place within the granite itself. Then, just at the conclusion of the puja, the rains began again and showered the region for yet another two weeks. It was more rain than the region had received in many years. In Yoga, rain is considered a great blessing from the divine, for with it, crops flourish and people are nourished.

"The temple is built to last for thousands of years. The quality of granite holds up extremely well over the centuries. Although small, it is very artful and energetically magnificent. The tranquility of the grounds is amazing. Scenes from Babaji's life are depicted in granite reliefs around the top of the temple.

"His Early Years

"Babaji has revealed that he was kidnapped at an early age from his hometown and taken to North India to be sold into slavery. In present-day Kolkata, he was purchased and soon released, where he migrated to Varanasi. In due course, he mastered the principles of both Vedanta and Siddhanta, and pierced the barriers to understanding the Siddhas. Having reached the limitations of academic knowledge, he began an extensive pilgrimage and course of sadhana. From the coast of Bengal, he undertook a pilgrimage by boat to the site of the Kali temple in Chittagong and also the powerful Chittagong Hill in Bangladesh. There, following intense sadhana, he had daily exchanges with Maa Kali and became intimate with her majesty, power and grace, mastering the path of Kaula Marg Tantra. He experienced Kali very tangibly in all her sixty-four emanations (sixty-four Yoginis). Later, Babaji influenced other Siddhas like Vashistha and Macchendranath (Macchamuni), who elevated Kaula Marg Tantra to a grand tradition. This led to the construction of sixty-four Yogini temples, mostly in North India. That hill, where Babaji performed tapas, later became a Bhavani Shakti temple and, in later centuries, identified as one of the celebrated fifty-two Shakti Peeths, or vortex shrines of Devi. It seems that he returned to that hill temple in later centuries. The Maha Kali Chew Mantra is the connection between Kali and Babaji.

"Returning to Kolkata, Babaji sailed to Katirgama, Sri Lanka, where he ultimately experienced Nirvakalpa Samadhi, the breathless state of God and Truth union. In doing so, he reestablished an ancient and powerful link with the eighteen Siddhas, particularly the scientific Siddha, Bogar.

"Coutrallam Falls in Tamil Nadu is the site where Babaji was initiated into Kriya by the great Siddha Agasthya.

"Babaji then journeyed to Coutrallam in Tamil Nadu, where he was initiated into Kriya by another of the eighteen Siddhas, Sage Agasthya. He then migrated to a cave in the high Himalayas and performed tapas for five years.

In the process, the very atoms of his physical body were permeated with and transformed by divine light-vibration. From that point on, he had no shadow and he had no footprint.

"His dynamic second cousin, Mataji, soon joined him and following his lead, attained a similar state, the golden deathless body of Soruba Samadhi. Yogananda introduced Mataji as Babaji's sister or cousin-sister, a common term of endearment in Indian culture. Yogi Ramaiah, who also spent time with Babaji in the physical body, explained a different reality than that. Let there be no ambiguity about the relationship between Babaji and Mataji. Yogiar many times confirmed that Babaji and Mataji were in a Shiva-Shakti union. Babaji and Mataji worked through the sixty-four Tantric Kriyas without a fall. Thus, having mastered the paths of Vedanta, Siddhantha, and Kaula Marg Tantra together, Mataji ascended into her predestined avatarship.

"Babaji in Our Current Era

> *"The breath that arose 12 matras long; if you can control and absorb within, well may you live a thousand years on land and sea; for the body, perishes not.'*
>
> "Thirumandiram V722

"High in the remote rocky mountains of the Kumoan Himalayas, the eternal Babaji lives today, as he has for millennia, retaining his physical form only for the benefit of humanity. It has long been understood that those who descend from the celestial realm (*avatars*) often bring with them outward signs of their inward freedom. Thus, there have been other Avatars that cast no shadow or footprint. There are others as well who have breathed life into a corpse or instantly moved through time and space with impunity. There have been others too, who lived without food or drink, who walked upon water, or moved upon air. But few are they whose physical form, manifesting the golden light of immortality, does not decay or age. And few indeed are they who can move through the physical world with mastery of every plane of existence, fully active and yet with breathing and mind perfectly stilled. Babaji reigns supreme as the great avatar of Vedanta, Siddhantha, and Kaula Marg Tantra. He is at the headwaters of all the sacred tributaries of Yoga and Tantra. From him has emerged every stream of Kriya itself and his guiding hand is ever present.

"He is seen and recognized only by those whom he chooses. Although he has appeared in many forms over the centuries, he frequently manifests as a timeless youth. His black hair is aflame with copper-golden rays of light-energy and his well-toned body reflects that of an athletic youth. His dark eyes, awash with light and love, penetrate the soul. His countenance is surrounded with authority and mystery. He is approachable and seen only by those of purified consciousness. He is known as the great yogi, the ancient youth of sixteen summers, as he attained immortality at a young age. His presence is not frightening at all, as some have thought. His presence is massively calming. In his presence one can think only what he allows. It is impossible to approach him without his inward permission. He is the great guiding father who was the loving guide behind all one's earthly fathers in every lifetime.

"Who is this great mysterious yogi who cannot be reduced to a rule? Like the cosmic Lord, he manifests the form and energy held dear by the devotee, nor can any mortal reduce him to a rule. The stellar star of his attainment is impossible for the mortal mind to comprehend. He is both multicultural and multi-linguistic and demonstrates a freedom from any limit. Every aspect of his remarkable life reflects this freedom. Miraculous stories of his life, including bringing the dead to life, manifest multiple bodies at the same time, and the ability to appear and disappear at will abound. He is so much more than an astral being, limited to a ghost body. He manifests a physical body with toes that have form and substance like a human being, except that they project light, fragrance and bliss when touched.

"In 1888 Madam Blavatsky, founder of the Theosophical Society, described Babaji in her great treatise, the 'Secret Doctrine,' as follows: 'It is He who changes form, yet remains ever the same, and it is He, again, who holds spiritual sway over the initiated adepts throughout the world. He is, as said, the nameless one who has so many names and yet, whose names and very nature are unknown. He is THE INITIATOR, called the GREAT SACRIFICE for sitting at the threshold of Light, He looks into it from within the circle of darkness, which He will not cross, nor will He quit His post until the last day of this lifecycle. Why does the solitary watcher remain at His self-chosen post? Why does He sit by the fountain of primeval wisdom, of which He drinks no longer, for He has naught to learn what He does not know—aye, neither on this earth nor in its heaven? Because the lonely sore-footed pilgrims, on their journey back to their home, are never sure till the last moment of not losing their way, in this limitless desert of illusion and matter called earth-life. Because He would show the way to that region of freedom and light from which He is a voluntary exile himself, to every prisoner who has succeeded in liberating himself from the bonds of flesh and illusion. Because, in short, He has sacrificed Himself for the sake of mankind, though but few selected may profit by the great sacrifice.

"Babaji as a Tantric

"Many people are aware of Babaji's contribution to Yoga and Kriya. Few, however, are aware of his achievements as a tantric master, along the lines of the Siddha Macchindranath. The Tamil Tantric, Rudranath Giri Maharaj, has revealed that Babaji is the avatar of great sacrifice for the emerging golden age of Kriya and that his glorious Shakti, taking form as Bhairavi, has regenerated the Kaula Marg tantric path as well, for the benefit and spiritual growth of all humanity. For Babaji and Mataji, a hundred years is but a day. Together they performed dynamic tantra sadhana in a small triangular cave near Gangotri. They have always worked quietly behind the scenes. Thousands of world and spiritual leaders are influenced by their 'tapas' at critical times, although most in an unconscious way. They seek absolutely no acknowledgment as they guide many toward spiritual awakening. They work on all planes and are literally 'a bridge for those who seek the farther shore.' A siddha in the ultimate sense is one who has attained perfection in all planes, including the physical. As defined in the Upanishads, a siddha is one who has progressed from the exalted state of freed while living (jivan mukta) to supremely free with full power over death (para mukta). This state is referred to in the Siddhantha tradition as soruba mukti, or soruba samadhi.

"Babaji Speaks

"Who is Babaji? Like God himself, he morphs into the forms that the devotee holds dear. He resides in the formless forms as well, such as the great tradition of Monism expounded by Adi Shankaracharya (whom he initiated).Speaking in ecstasy, Babaji once demonstrated his mastery of the Advaita Vedanta path as he literally described his consciousness to his chosen disciples, V.T.N. and Yo- giar, as follows:

> *'"I am existence-knowledge-bliss absolute. I am the absolute and supreme Self, both within and without the finitude. I am truth,*

eternal and everlasting. I am the only one, all in myself: None exist save I, in and through all that exists. I am ever all-existence itself. I am the changeless one in the midst of all changes. I am the formless in all forms...I am the living ocean of ecstasy that rages wild and surges and storms and levels down the earth and heavens. I beat in every breast, see in every eye, throb in every pulse, smile in every flower, shine in the lightning and roar in the thunder. I flutter in the leaves, I hiss in the winds, and I roll in the surging seas. I am the wisdom of the wise, the strength of the strong, the heroism of the heroic. I am the impersonal personality of the whole universe. I am the infinite, the eternal, and the immortal Self. Truth flows from me just as light radiates from the sun and fragrance emanates from a flower on the immutable and indescribable Atman, the dynamic principle of existence and the infinite ocean of everlasting conciseness.'

"Our prayer

"Babaji, you are our light and guide. Awaken us from the slumber of the ages. Please guide every thought, every action, every desire toward purity and light. Humble us, that we may be receptive to your Grace. Above all, shepherd us through the transition at the end of each life with a firm but kind hand that we may reside eternally at your lotus feet and serve the light forever. May Atman alone dominate the consciousness! May the power and majesty of your light and love manifest in every plane and every cell. Let the akashic record reflect that we lived nobly in each moment."

I took a break and took a sip of coffee and a couple of cookies.

"What an amazing divine personality," said Madhu.

Jagadguru Ramanandacharya Rajivlochanacharya

"I will now speak about another divine personality, Jagadguru Ramanancharya Rajivlochanacharya, my revered Guruji.

"Guruji became a Jagadguru at the age of thirty-six years at the Maha Kumbha Mela in Haridwar in 1998, the youngest after Adi Shankaracharya, centuries before at the age of thirty-two years.

"The elevation to the position of Jagadguru starts from a Sadhu to a Swami (Mandaleshwar) to a Maha Mandaleshwar. One out of 108, Maha Mandaleshwar is elevated to the title of Acharya Maha Mandaleshwar and one out of 108

Acharya Maha Mandaleshwars is given the honor and title of Jagadguru by the entire community of saints of India. To achieve this by thirty-six years is nothing short of extraordinary. Jagadguru's divinity took roots even before birth. His parents went to Lord Jagannath's temple in Orissa, India, to pray for a son after they were blessed earlier with daughters. Guruji was born after that.

"Through the years Guruji rose above the sense-gratifying forces to carry on his mission of spreading peace, love and compassion for all humanity with the sacrosanct system of OM Kriya Yoga, which he was initiated into by Mahavatar Kriya Babaji in the Himalayas earlier.

"This system of Kriya Yoga was taught by Lord Krishna to Prince Arjuna in the Bhagavad Gita. It is a system of using the Brahmanada 'OM,' or the primordial sound, and kriyas to awaken the Kundalini in us. It helps to awaken the cosmic energy in us and elevate our consciousness to the divine level.

"Guruji was directed by Mahavatar Kriya Babaji in Mount Kailash in 1995 to teach the science of self-realization to people irrespective of their nationality, caste, creed, religion or gender and help them drink the divine nectar of God's love.

"Guruji had created the OM Kriya Yantra according to his realizations. Ishwar, God, is the Supreme Being; Sadhana, the discipline of life; Karma, the rightful duties; Love, essence of God; Seva, egoless and selfless service; and Meditation, concentration of mind.

"Guruji travelled to Trinidad and Tobago for a Ramayana Conference on an invitation from the President of Trinidad and Tobago. He has travelled to USA, Holland, UK, South Africa, among other countries, to spread OM Kriya Yoga."

I stopped to sip on my coffee and replenish my energies with a couple of cookies.

"Is he still alive? He is young. May I meet him?" Madhu asked.

"Unfortunately, he is not in the world of living, from what we know. He left his body at the age of forty-one years in Mansarovar on Shivaratri night in meditation," I said with extreme sadness.

"Why do good people leave so early? The bad ones have long lives," Madhu said with indignation.

"At times that is the cosmic rule. These great souls are required in other worlds to do higher work and also, they find it difficult to withstand the vibrations of the people of this planet," I remarked.

"Madhu, let us hear about the Kailash Temple," I said with eagerness.

[40]"One of my amazing experiences was visiting the Kailash Temple. The Kailasha, or Kailashanatha, temple is the largest of the rock-cut Hindu temples at the Ellora Caves, Aurangabad District, Maharashtra, India. A megalith carved from a rock cliff face, it is considered one of the most remarkable cave temples in the world because of its size, architecture and sculptural treatment, and 'the climax of the rock-cut phase of Indian architecture.' The top of the superstructure over the sanctuary is 32.6 meters (107 feet) above the level of the court below, although the rock face slopes downwards from the rear of the temple to the front. Archaeologists believe it is made from a single rock.

"The Kailasa temple (Cave 16) is the largest of the thirty-four Buddhist, Jain and Hindu cave temples and monasteries known collectively as the Ellora Caves, ranging for over two kilometers (1.2 miles) along the sloping basalt cliff at the site. Most of the excavation of the temple is generally attributed to the eighth-century Rashtrakuta king, Krishna I (r. c. 756–773), with some elements completed later. The temple architecture shows traces of Pallava and Chalukya styles. The temple contains a number of relief and free-standing sculptures on a grand scale equal to the architecture, though only traces remain of the paintings that originally decorated it.

"Kailasa temple lacks a dedicatory inscription, but there is no doubt that it was commissioned by a Rashtrakuta ruler. Its construction is generally attributed to the Rashtrakuta king Krishna I (r. 756-773 C.E.), based on two epigraphs that link the temple to 'Krishnaraja.'

The Kailasa Temple is notable for its *vertical* excavation—carvers started at the top of the original rock and excavated downward. The traditional methods were rigidly followed by the master architect, which could not have been achieved by excavating from the front.

"The Kailasa temple architecture is different from the earlier style prevalent in the Deccan region. As stated above, it appears to be based on the Virupaksha Temple at Pattadakal and the Kailasa temple at Kanchi, but it is not an exact imitation of these two temples. The southern influence on the temple architecture can be attributed to the involvement of Chalukya and Pallava artists in its construction. The indigenous Deccan artisans appear to have played a subordinate role in the temple's construction.

---

[40] *Incredibleindia.org.*

"The entrance to the temple courtyard features a low gopuram. Most of the deities at the left of the entrance are Shaivaite (affiliated with Shiva) while on the righthand side the deities are Vaishnavaites (affiliated with Vishnu). A two-storied gateway opens to reveal a U-shaped courtyard. The dimensions of the courtyard are 82 meters by 46 meters at the base. The courtyard is edged by a columned arcade three stories high. The arcades are punctuated by huge sculpted panels, and alcoves containing enormous sculptures of a variety of deities. Originally, flying bridges of stone connected these galleries to central temple structures, but these have fallen. Some of the most famous sculptures are Shiva the ascetic, Shiva the dancer, Shiva being warned by Parvati about the demon Ravana, and the river goddess.

"Within the courtyard, there is a central shrine dedicated to Shiva, and an image of his mount Nandi (the sacred bull). The central shrine housing the lingam features a flat-roofed mandapa supported by sixteen pillars, and a Dravidian shikhara. The shrine—complete with pillars, windows, inner and outer rooms, gathering halls, and an enormous stone lingam at its heart— is carved with niches, plasters, windows as well as images of deities, *mithunas* (erotic male and female figures) and other figures. As is traditional in Shiva temples, Nandi sits on a porch in front of the central temple. The Nandi mandapa and main Shiva temple are each about 7 meters high, and built on two stories. The lower stories of the Nandi Mandapa are both solid structures, decorated with elaborate illustrative carvings. The base of the temple has been carved to suggest that elephants are holding the structure aloft. A rock bridge connects the Nandi Mandapa to the porch of the temple. The base of the temple hall features scenes from Mahabharata and Ramayana."

Madhu calmly took a sip of his coffee and turned to me and said, "Shomikda, can you imagine the brilliance of the artisans in creating this wonder of the world so many centuries ago, allegedly with minimum sophisticated equipment and labor? I somehow feel there is something beyond this narrative."

I nodded to accept and appreciate his train of thoughts.

"Also, why do you think many temples of India have erotic figures of men and women?" he asked.

"I believe that there are two reasons. One is so that impure-minded people, spirits and other beings will not enter the pure sanctum of the temple.

They would be stuck seeing the figures on the wall of the temple. Only the pure-minded people will enter the holy sanctum.

"The other reason might be because in olden times, the human being was not looked at with despise in certain aspects. Sex is as much a part of human life and anything else. It is depicted naturally as part of life. When the Europeans came, they imposed their sense of morality on us and termed these sculptures as dirty or erotic," I said, thinking deeply.

Evening was setting in and Madhu decided to call it a day. He moved toward the door and I reached him with a friendly hug to express our feelings of friendship.

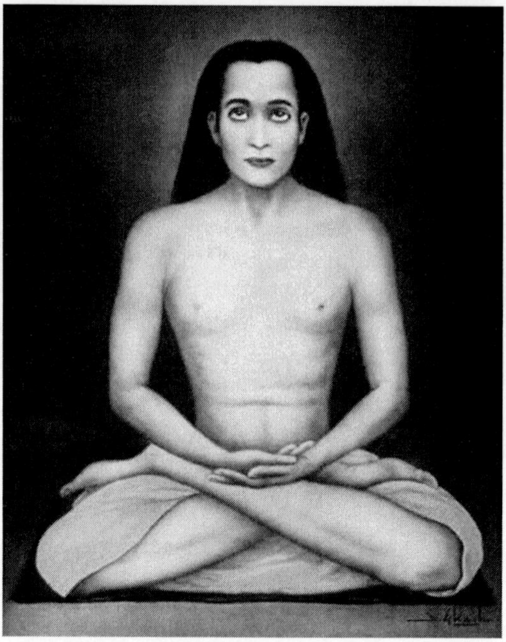

Mahavatar Kriya Babaji. Credit: Shrine of the Masters at Ananda Village

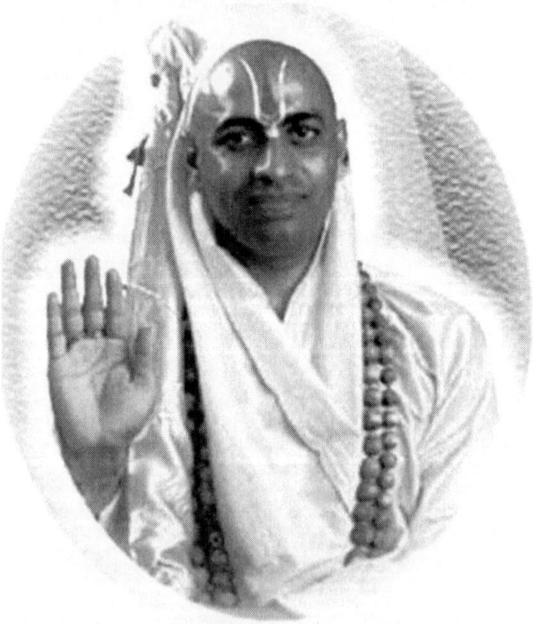

Jagadguru Ramanandacharya Rajivlochanacharya (Guruji). Credit: OKYF

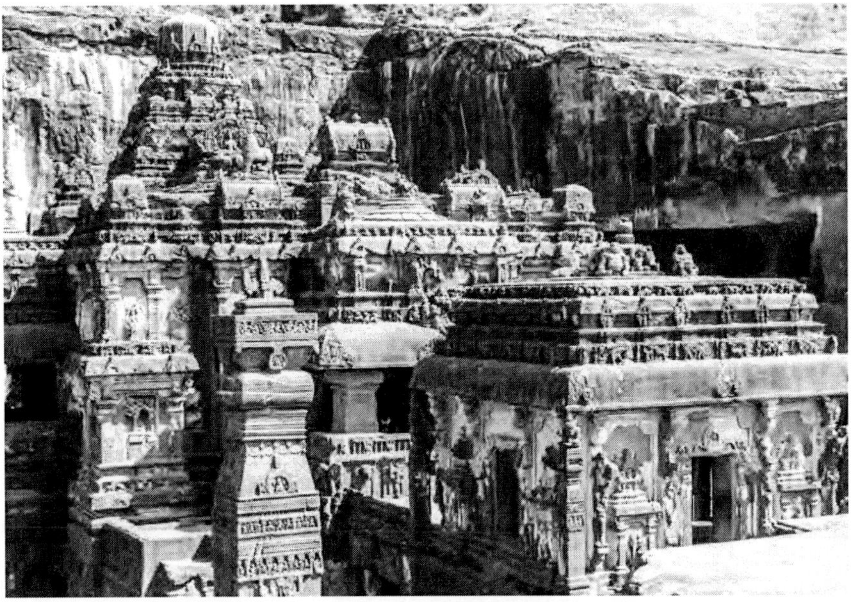

Kailasha Temple in Ellora, Maharashtra. Credit: mathess

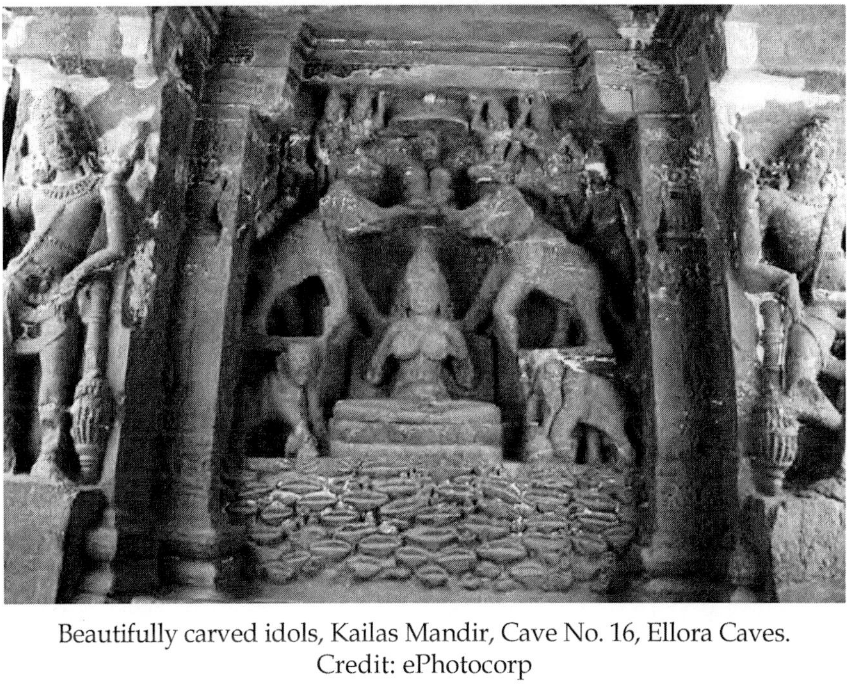

Beautifully carved idols, Kailas Mandir, Cave No. 16, Ellora Caves.
Credit: ePhotocorp

Chapter 12

Leading a Balanced Life

Madhu had come to my house one weekend and we started discussing leading a balanced life.

He said, "Shomikda, tell me something about leading a balanced life. People will be in a dilemma as to whether they should renounce the world and meditate and look for self-realization or lead a householder's life."

I started, [41]"Hindu life is lived in a balanced manner. The Purusharthas, which literally mean an 'object of human pursuit,' is a key concept in Hinduism, and refers to the four proper goals or aims of a human life. The four Purusharthas are Dharma (righteousness, moral values), Artha (prosperity, economic values), Kama (pleasure, love, psychological values) and Moksha (liberation, spiritual values). All four Purusharthas are important, but in cases of conflict, Dharma is considered more important than Artha or Kama in Hindu philosophy. Moksha is considered the ultimate ideal of human life. At the same time, this is not a consensus among all Hindus, and many have different interpretations of the hierarchy, and even as to whether one should exist. Historical Indian scholars recognized and debated the inherent tension between active pursuit of wealth (Artha purusartha) and pleasure (Kama), and renunciation of all wealth and pleasure for the sake of spiritual liberation (Moksha).

"Let us explore the significance of each:

---

[41] *https://timesofindia.indiatimes.com/readersblog/leading-a-balanced-life-though-pursuit-of-purushartha/leading-a-balanced-life-though-pursuit-of-puru-shartha-12089/.*

- Dharma: represents behaviors that are considered to be in accord with *rta*, the order that makes life and universe possible, and includes duties, rights, laws, conduct, virtues and *right way of living*. Hindu Dharma includes the religious duties, moral rights and duties of each individual as well as behaviors that enable social order, right conduct, and those that are virtuous. Dharma is that which all existing beings must accept and respect to sustain harmony and order in the world.
- Artha: signifies the "means of life," activities and resources that enable one to be in a state one wants to be in. *Artha* incorporates wealth, career, activity to make a living, financial security and economic prosperity. The proper pursuit of Artha is considered an important aim of human life in Indian culture.
- Kama: signifies desire, wish, passion, emotions, pleasure of the senses, the aesthetic enjoyment of life, affection, or love, with or without sexual connotations. Kāma is 'love' without violating Dharma (moral responsibility), Artha (material prosperity) and one's journey toward Moksha (spiritual liberation).
- Moksha: signifies emancipation, liberation or release. In some schools of Hinduism, *Moksha* connotes freedom from *saṃsāra*, the cycle of death and rebirth; in other schools Moksha connotes freedom, self-knowledge, self-realization and liberation in this life.

"Ancient Indian literature emphasizes that Dharma is foremost. If Dharma is ignored, Artha and Kama—profit and pleasure, respectively—lead to social chaos. The Gautama Dharmashastra, Apastamba Dharmasutra and Yājñavalkya Smṛti, as examples, all suggest that Dharma comes first and is more important than Artha and Kama.

"Kama states the relative value of three goals as follows: Artha is more important and should precede Kama, while Dharma is more important and should precede both Kama and Artha. Kautiliya's Arthashastra, however, argues that Artha is the foundation for the other two. Without prosperity and security in society or at individual level, both moral life and sensuality become difficult. Poverty breeds vice and hate, while prosperity breeds virtues and love, suggested Kautiliya. Kautilya adds that all three are mutually connected, and one should not cease enjoying life, nor virtuous behavior, nor pursuit of wealth creation. Excessive pursuit of any one aspect of life with complete rejection of other two harms all three, including the one excessively pursued. The sastras observe that the relative precedence of Artha, Kama and Dharma are naturally different with age.

"Moksha is considered in Hinduism as the *parama-puruṣārtha,* or ultimate goal of human life.

"For the balance in life to be maintained, we need to remember and follow Patanjali's Yoga Sutras:

1. Physical health: Physical health is very important to lead a balanced life. Asana, pranayama are very important in keeping the body healthy.
2. Mental health: For the mind to be at peace and happy, practice meditation, detachment from technology and rat race for a while.
3. Emotional health: To maintain a good emotional state of health, you need to learn to relax, induce happiness inside you, develop gratitude for everything, listen to good music, among other activities.
4. Spiritual health: Developing a sense of gratitude, connect with your inner self, create a loving relationship with God and pray to Him.
5. Social health: Connecting well with people around you—your family, friends, coworkers and others. Helping others is also a very important part of creating a healthy social environment. Maintain association with like-minded good people.
6. Environmental health: Maintaining the environment is very important in today's world. Being responsible for clean and unpolluted environment is a must. Saving the planet from plastic pollution and other pollution is a must to save the earth for the succeeding generations.
7. Work-related health: It is necessary to maintain good relations with colleagues in the office or business, whatever you do. Maintaining a work-life balance is a must for a balanced life. As a leader you should always train yourself more and more and also lift up others through training, mentoring and encouragement.
8. Financial health: Maintaining financial health is very important in maintaining a balance in life. Financial investments, savings, wealth creation all go a long way to create balance in life. Proper financial

management helps a stress-free mind, more time to have a work-life balance and enables a quality of life that is necessary to lead a good life.

"From the above study, it is clear that leading a balanced life involves internal and external factors.

"Internal (Mind, Heart, Health)

- Mind: Challenging oneself intellectually vs. creating opportunities for your mind to rest
- Heart: Giving love vs. receiving love
- Health: Eating, drinking, and exercising properly vs. resting and treating yourself to some extra yummies

"External (Work, Social, Family, Fun)

- Work: Pushing yourself to achieve goals vs. seeing the bigger picture and enjoying the ride
- Social: Satisfying your social desires vs. taking time for yourself
- Family: Fulfilling your familial responsibilities vs. creating healthy boundaries
- Fun: Giving time for things that you enjoy doing vs. ensuring you don't overdo it

"Maintaining balance can be difficult but trying to be great at everything and accomplish it all at once is just not possible. Yes, we all have things we have to do. Many of us have to go to work or school. We also have to eat and sleep. We all have responsibilities. Balance is about marrying the 'must-dos' with the 'need-to-dos,' like building relationships, taking care of our physical and mental wellbeing, and letting the rest go without beating ourselves up about it.

"Balance isn't passive; it's not just happening for you if you do not have any intent about it. We often use images of women in relaxing poses to visualize 'balance,' and while adding in that practice may be a byproduct of what balance looks like to you, understand that it takes active mental participation to get you there. You need to first believe that you deserve balance and then set an intentional course to get you there.

"Whether you are a housewife, or have a career woman alongside motherhood, it is most difficult. Creating balance is not about perfection; it's about building everyday habits that honor your body both physically and mentally. "When you are able to lead a balanced life, you experience deep, restful sleep; have more energy, vitality, and mental clarity; shed excess weight that doesn't belong to you; and find an inner calm even when life is chaotic. So lead a balanced life from the lessons of ancient India as well as modern suggestions."

"That was a very good starter for leading a balanced life," said Madhu.

"Let me talk about the Jagannath Temple of Puri, where I had visited," he began.[42]"Odisha is known as the land of Lord Jagannath (literally meaning the Lord of the Universe). The temple built in the 12th Century A.D. has been the epicenter of Jagannath cult and sees pilgrims flocking the temple town of Puri from all corners of the world throughout the year.

"The mysticism associated with the cult of Lord Jagannath overshadows the architectural brilliance of this magnificent temple. Built on a raised platform, the gigantic temple is an architectural marvel in its own right.

"The temple saw new additions to its structure till about the 16th Century A.D. Unlike other temples of the region, the carvings on the temples are predominantly of gods and goddesses. The entire temple complex is enclosed within two concentric walls, the Kuruma Bheda (inner wall) and the Meghnad Pachira (wall). The main entrance to the temple is through Singhadwara, located on the Eastern front of the temple with three other entrances along the four cardinal directions. However, these are not architecturally aligned, indicating that the other entrances might have been created for security purposes since the temple was at the eye of the storm during the tumultuous period between the 16th and 18th centuries.

"Some of the architectural feats of the temple

"The main temple is constructed in such a way that no shadow of the temple falls on the ground at any time of the day.

"The huge temple complex covers an area of over 400,000 square feet (37,000 miles^2) and is surrounded by a high fortified wall. This 20-foot-(6.1-

[42] *https://odishatourism.gov.in/content/tourism/en/discover/attractions/temples-monuments/jagannath-temple.html.*

meter)-high wall is known as Meghanada Pacheri. Another wall, known as kurma bedha, surrounds the main temple. It contains at least 120 temples and shrines. With its sculptural richness and fluidity of the Oriya style of temple architecture, it is one of the most magnificent monuments of India. The temple has four distinct sectional structures, namely:

1. Deula, Vimana or Garba griha (Sanctum sanctorum), where the triad deities are lodged on the ratnavedi (Throne of Pearls). In Rekha Deula style;
2. Mukhashala (Frontal porch);
3. Nata mandir/Natamandapa, which is also known as the Jagamohan (Audience Hall/Dancing Hall); and
4. Bhoga Mandapa (Offerings Hall).

The main temple is a curvilinear temple and crowning the top is the 'Neelachakra' (an eight-spoked wheel) of Lord Vishnu. It is made out of Ashtadhatu and is considered sacrosanct. Among the existing temples in Orissa, the temple of Shri Jagannath is the highest. The temple tower was built on a raised platform of stone and, rising to 214 feet (65 meters) above the inner sanctum where the deities reside, dominates the surrounding landscape. The pyramidal roofs of the surrounding temples and adjoining halls, or mandapas, rise in steps toward the tower like a ridge of mountain peaks.

"The Nilachakra, or the blue wheel, perched on top of the temple, is made of eight metals, or asta dhatu. It is believed that if you see the Nilachakra, it is as good as seeing the Lord himself.

The flag, or the Patitapabana, flows in the opposite direction of the wind and is changed every day at sunset. The feat of changing the flag's rests with a family appointed by the king. They have been doing this ritual for over eight hundred years, climbing 165 meters, bare feet without any support.

"The Mahaprasad, or the offering to the Lord, is prepared on fire lit by wood charcoal and rice and vegetables, cereals, etc., are put in earthen pots and placed on the fire, one on top of the other. The pot on the top cooks first.

"The Aruna stambha: The 33-foot monolith structure pillar in front of the Singhadwar, or the main entrance of the temple, was originally located at the Sun Temple, Konark.

"Another unique feature of the temple is that the idols of the holy trinity are carved out of wood rather than stone or metal idols. They are also the only deity with the trappings of mortality. Jagannath, Balabhadra and Subhadra are a trio of deities worshipped at the temple. The inner sanctum of the temple contains the deities of them carved from sacred neem logs known as *daru*, sitting on the bejeweled platform or *ratnabedi*, along with deities of Sudarshana Chakra, Madanmohan, Sridevi and Vishwadhatri. The deities are adorned with different clothing and jewels according to the season. Worship of these deities predates the building of the temple and may have originated in an ancient tribal shrine.

"Festivals

"There are many festivals and rituals associated with the Lord; we list a couple.

> "**Devasnana Purnima**: The annual bathing ritual, where the holy trinity has been brought out from their sanctum and seated in a raised platform and bathed with purified water drawn from a well within the temple premises.
>
> "**Chariot Festival**: This happens during the month of June/July. During the festival, the Lord comes out to the street to greet his devotees, people irrespective of caste, creed and color can seek his blessings. The Jagannath, Subhadra and Balaram are usually worshiped in the sanctum of the temple at Puri, but once during the month of Asadha (Rainy Season of Orissa, usually falling in month of June or July), they are brought out onto the Bada Danda (main street of Puri) and travel three kilometers to the Shri Gundicha Temple, in huge chariots (ratha), allowing the public to have darshan. This festival is known as Rath Yatra, meaning the journey (yatra) of the chariots (ratha). The Rathas are huge wheeled wooden structures, which are built anew every year and are pulled by the devotees. The chariot for Jagannath is approximately 45 feet high and 35 feet square and takes about two months to construct. The artists and painters of Puri decorate the cars and paint flower petals and other designs on the wheels, the wood-carved charioteer and horses, and the inverted lotuses on the wall behind the throne. The huge chariots of Jagannath pulled during Rath Yatra is the etymological origin of the English word 'Juggernaut.'

"The most significant ritual associated with the Ratha-Yatra is the *chhera pahara*. During the festival, the Gajapati King wears the outfit of a sweeper and sweeps all around the deities and chariots in the *Chera Pahara* (sweeping with water) ritual. The Gajapati King cleanses the road before the chariots with a gold-handled broom and sprinkles sandalwood water and powder with utmost devotion. As per the custom, although the Gajapati King has been considered the most exalted person in the Kalingan kingdom, he still renders the menial service to Jagannath. This ritual signified that under the lordship of Jagannath, there is no distinction between the powerful sovereign Gajapati King and the most humble devotee. *Chera pahara* is held on two days, on the first day of the Ratha Yatra, when the deities are taken to garden house at Mausi Maa Temple, and again on the last day of the festival, when the deities are ceremoniously brought back to the Shri Mandir.

"As per another ritual, the deities are taken out from the Shri Mandir to the Chariots in *Pahandi vijay*.

"In the Ratha Yatra, the three deities are taken from the Jagannath Temple in the chariots to the Gundicha Temple, where they stay for nine days. Thereafter, the deities again ride the chariots back to Shri Mandir in *bahuda yatra*. On the way back, the three chariots halt at the Mausi Maa Temple and the deities are offered *Poda Pitha,* a kind of baked cake thatis generally consumed by the Odisha people only.

"The observance of the Rath Yatra of Jagannath dates back to the period of the Puranas. Vivid descriptions of this festival are found in Brahma Purana, Padma Purana, and Skanda Purana. Kapila Samhita also refers to Rath Yatra. In Moghul period also, King Ramsingh of Jaipur, Rajasthan, has been described as organizing the Rath Yatra in the 18th century. In Orissa, kings of Mayurbhanj and Parlakhemundi were organizing the Rath Yatra, though the most grand festival in terms of scale and popularity takes place at Puri.

"It is noted by Western scholars that the ruling Ganga dynasty instituted the Rath Yatra at the completion of the great temple around 1150 A.D. This festival was one of those Hindu festivals that was reported to the Western world very early."

Madhu sat quietly for some time.

I said, "I have been to the Jagannath Temple twice in my life. Amazing spiritual experience. Beautiful architecture and remarkable, miraculous features."

We both parted ways for the day and looked forward to our next meeting.

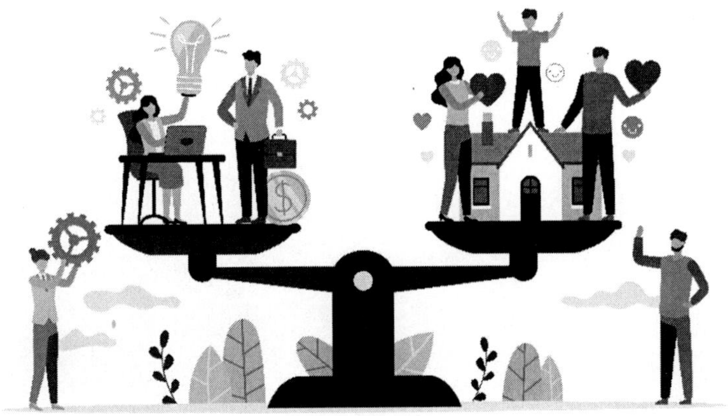

Home, work and self-development on scales.
Credit: Tetiana Lazunova

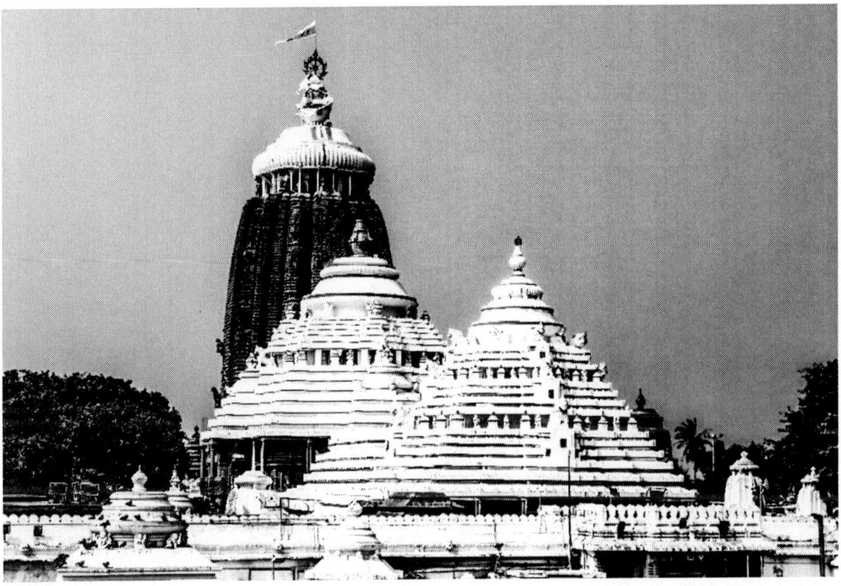

The Sri Jagannatha Temple is an important Hindu temple dedicated to Lord Jagannatha, a form of Lord Vishnu, located on the eastern coast of India at Puri, Odisha. Credit: Kali Justine

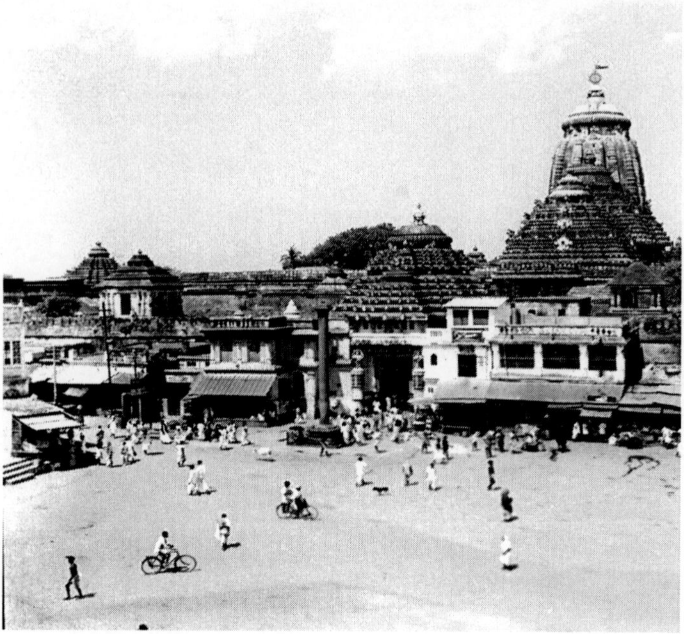

Entrance to Jagannath Temple Puri. Credit: Ministry of External Affairs, Government of India

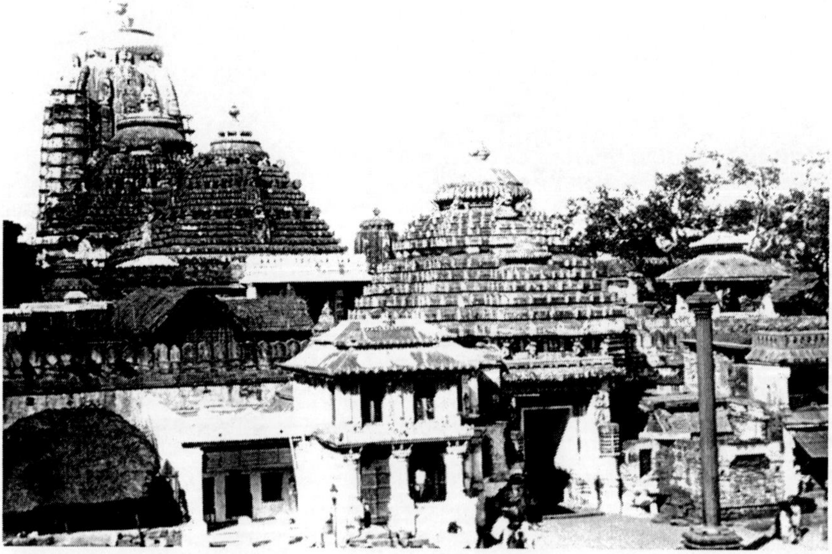

Jagannath Temple, Puri. Credit: Ministry of External Affairs, Government of India

Chapter 13

Realizing the Oneness amongst Everything

It was another weekend day. Madhu and I sat on our sofas at my home with coffee and samosas served by my dear wife.

"Shomikda, I have heard so much about spirituality from you. Why do people not see the oneness amongst us and unite as humanity?" Madhu asked in between taking a couple of sips from his cup of coffee.

"Madhu, it is a work in progress for everyone. It is a process. This kind of realization does not happen in one day. It takes years, a lifetime and even many lives. But the important thing is to progress on that path. Move slowly but surely on that path.

"It starts at the time the child is in the womb. The mother, especially, needs to read spiritual books and practice spiritual practices that help the child imbibe those values form the womb. When the child is born, then both the parents should help the child inculcate spiritual values to enable them to grow up in a healthy environment for spiritual growth.

"The next stage involves the introduction of Yoga from the Yoga Sutras of Patanjali. Let me remind you once again.

"Yama

"*Yama* is social behavior, how you treat others and the world around you. These are moral principles. Sometimes they are called the 'don'ts' or the 'thou shalt nots.' There are five yamas:

- **Nonviolence** (*ahimsa*). Do no harm to any creature in thought or deed. But you have the right to defend yourself.

- **Truth and honesty** (*satya*). Tell no lies. Cheating in business deals falls into this category.
- **Nonstealing** (*asteya*). Do not steal material objects (a jewel) or intangibles such as the center of attention or your child's chance to learn responsibility or independence by doing something on his own.
- **Nonlust** (*brahmacharya*). Don't worry; this is not a call to celibacy. Many yogis of old were married and had families of their own. The person who practices brahmacharya avoids meaningless sexual encounters and sees divinity in all.
- **Nonpossessiveness** (*aparigraha*). Free yourself from greed, hoarding, and collecting. Do you really need more shirts, another car, or to take over the conversation every time you see your friends? Make your life as simple as possible.

"Niyama

"*Niyama* is inner discipline and responsibility, how we treat ourselves. These are sometimes called observances, the 'do's' or the 'thou shalts.' There are five niyamas:

- **Purity** (*shauca*). Purity is achieved through the practice of the five yamas, which help clear away the negative physical and mental states of being. Keep yourself, your clothing, and your surroundings clean. Eat fresh and healthy food. The next time you joke about treating your body like a temple, think of this niyama.
- **Contentment** (*santosha*). Cultivate contentment and tranquility by finding happiness with what you have and who you are. Seek happiness in the moment, take responsibility for where you are, and choose to grow from there.
- **Austerity** (*tapas*). Show discipline in body, speech, and mind. The purpose of developing self-discipline is not to become ascetic, but to control and direct the mind and body for higher spiritual aims or purposes.
- **Study of the sacred text** (*svadhyaya*). Study sacred scriptures, which are whatever books are relevant to you and inspire and teach you. Education changes a person's outlook on life. As Yoga Master B.K.S.

Iyengar says, a person starts 'to realize that all creation is meant for *bhakti* (adoration) rather than for *bhoga* (enjoyment), that all creation is divine, that there is divinity within oneself and that the energy which moves him is the same that moves the entire universe.'

- **Living with an awareness of the Divine** (*ishvara-pranidhana*). Be devoted to God, or whatever you consider divine.

"Asana

'"The posture of Yoga is steady and easy,' Patanjali says. Patanjali compares this to resting like the cosmic serpent on the waters of infinity. Although Westerners often consider the practice of asana or postures as an exercise regimen or a way to stay fit, Patanjali and other ancient yogis used asana to prepare the body for meditation. To sit for a lengthy time in contemplation required a supple and cooperative body. If you are free of physical distractions—such as your foot going to sleep—and can control the body, you can also control the mind. Patanjali said, 'Posture is mastered by freeing the body and mind from tension and restlessness and meditating on the infinite.'

"Pranayama

"*Prana* is the life force or energy that exists everywhere and flows through each of us through the breath. *Pranayama* is the control of breath. The basic movements of pranayama are inhalation, retention of breath, and exhalation. 'The yogi's life is not measured by the number of days but by the number of his breaths,' says Iyengar. 'Therefore, he follows the proper rhythmic patterns of slow, deep breathing.' The practice of pranayama purifies and removes distractions from the mind, making it easier to concentrate and meditate.

"Pratyahara

"*Pratyahara* is withdrawal of the senses. Pratyahara occurs during meditation, breathing exercises, or the practice of Yoga postures—any time when you are directing your attention inward. Concentration, in the Yoga room or the boardroom, is a battle with distracting senses. When you master pratyahara, you are able to focus because you no longer feel the itch on your big toe or hear the mosquito buzzing by your ear or smell the pizza warming up in the microwave.

"Dharana

"Concentration, or *dharana,* involves teaching the mind to focus on one point or image. 'Concentration is binding thought in one place,' says Patanjali. The goal is to still the mind—gently pushing away unnecessary thoughts—by fixing your mind on some object such as a candle flame, a flower, or a mantra. In dharana, concentration is effortless. You know the mind is concentrating when there is no sense of time passing.

"Dhyana

"Uninterrupted meditation without an object is called *dhyana.* Concentration (dharana) leads to the state of meditation. The goal of meditation is not unconsciousness or nothingness. It is heightened awareness and oneness with the universe. How do you tell the difference between concentration and meditation? If there is awareness of distraction, you are only concentrating and not meditating. The calm achieved in meditation spills over into all aspects of your life—during a hectic day at work, shopping for groceries, coordinating the Diwali party at your child's school.

"Samadhi

"The ultimate goal of the eightfold path to Yoga is *samadhi,* or absolute bliss. This is pure contemplation, super-consciousness, in which you and the universe are one. Those who have achieved samadhi are enlightened. Paramahansa Yogananda, author of *An Autobiography of a Yogi,* called it the state of God-Union.

"The eight limbs work together: The first five steps—yama, niyama asana, pranayama, and pratyahara—are the preliminaries of Yoga and build the foundation for spiritual life. They are concerned with the body and the brain. The last three, which would not be possible without the previous steps, are concerned with reconditioning the mind. They help the yogi to attain enlightenment or the full realization of oneness with Spirit. Enlightenment lasts forever, while a flat tummy can disappear with a week of binging.

"This system will help us develop into a better human being with empathy toward all.

"Practicing OM Kriya Yoga intertwined with the Yoga as in the Yoga Sutras will enhance the upliftment of the human consciousness from a budding stage to a fully bloomed state. In yogic terms, when the kundalini rises from Ajna chakra and toward Sahasrar, then the artificial vivisections of the society dissolve away and you see everything as part of the one cosmos. Full realization comes at that stage, but the feeling of oneness starts from the very beginning. Love is the most important factor in people's lives and is the most important and probably the only factor that encompasses Creation and beyond.

"God is supreme bliss and that is our core too. We have been encompassed by material energy, which divides us into different entities, suffering, and all the related vices that are there. Once we are able to evolve our consciousness out of that limitation and division by seeking our cores, we will find that we were supreme bliss all the time. We had forgotten this basic truth about our existence. These processes will enable us to rediscover our core and our actual existence.

"Lord Krishna said in the Bhagavad Gita that He is in everything small or big and everything is in Him and He is beyond everything. So, there is nothing other than Krishna anywhere. Different philosophies state different ideas but this is my understanding. However, I realize this is a different ball game.

"My suggestion to everyone is to start NOW. No matter how old you are, advance the evolution of your consciousness from this time so that you can start from a better position in your next life to get to realizing yourself. Remember, no one is without hope and no one is hopeless. Remember, you are a child of God and your love, relationship and surrender to Him will help you to uplift yourself in life. He is eternally with us and loving us. We suffer because we forgot the relationship with God and we let karma overtake us. The level of happiness that you can experience all the time from within yourself is directly proportional to the evolution of consciousness that you have attained.

"Evolution itself is karma. God has given us the freedom to create our own karma, especially at the human level. It is our choice. So, we create our karma and when we mess up due to our choices, we accuse God of being unkind and malevolent.

"One way in which not to mess up is to have a purpose in life and to surrender to God, building up a relationship with him and to love him. You should be God loving and not God fearing. God is our eternal, nearest and dearest friend.

"So, follow the Yoga Sutras of Sage Patanjali and follow OM Kriya Yoga to raise yourself to be a better human being, one day at a time, and you will see the change in your consciousness. It will also help in your life in the material world in terms of quality of work, relationships, habits, happiness, being stoic, and being in a peaceful state of being.

"Then the process of realizing the oneness amongst everything will start evolving within you."

I sat back gorging on the fresh hot samosas brought by my wife. Lectures always make me hungry.

Madhu turned to me and said, "It should be our duty to get back to our core, or Godhead."

"It should be. The faster we realize that and start the process, the better for us," I said with conviction.

Madhu turned to me and said, "Indeed, Shomikda. Let me tell you also about an amazing visit that I had to Shri Vishwanath Temple of Varanasi.

[43]"Situated on the western bank of the holy River Ganges, Varanasi is the oldest surviving city of the world and the cultural capital of India. It is in the heart of this city that there stands in its fullest splendor the Kashi Vishwanath Temple, in which is enshrined the Jyotirlinga of Shiva, Vishweshwara, or Vishwanath. Here come millions from India and abroad to seek the blessing and spiritual peace with the darshan of this Jyotirlinga, which confers liberation from the bondages of Maya and the inexorable tangles of the world. A simple glimpse of the Jyotirlinga is a soul cleansing experience that transforms life and puts it on the path of knowledge and devotion. Vishweshwara Jyotirlinga has a very special and unique significance in the spiritual history of India. Tradition has it that the merits earned by the darshan of other jyotirlinga scattered in various parts of India accrue to devotee by a single visit to Kashi Vishwanath Temple.

"Deeply and intimately implanted in our minds, the Kashi Vishwanath Temple has been a living embodiment of our timeless cultural traditions and highest spiritual values. The Temple has been visited by all great saints: Adi Shankaracharya, Ramakrishna Paramhansa, Swami Vivekananda, Goswami Tulsidas, Maharshi Dayanand Saraswati, Guru Nanak and several other spiritual personalities. The Kashi Vishwanath Temple attracts visitors from India and abroad as well and thereby symbolizes man's desire to live in peace and harmony with one another. Vishwanath being a supreme repository of this spiri-

[43] *https://shrikashivishwanath.org/.*

tual truth thus strengthens the bonds of universal brotherhood and fellow feeling at the national as well as international levels.

"On January 28, 1983, the temple was taken over by the Govt. of Uttar Pradesh and its management ever since stands entrusted to a Trust, with former Kashi Naresh as President and an Executive Committee with Divisional Commissioner as Chairman. The Temple in the present shape was built way back in 1780 by Late Maharani Ahilya Bai Holkar of Indore. In the year 1785 a Naubatkhana was built up in front of the Temple by the then-collector Mohd Ibrahim Khan at the instance of Governor General Warren Hastings. In 1839, the two domes of the Temple were covered by gold donated by Punjab Kesari Maharaja Ranjit Singh. Third dome still remains uncovered, Ministry of Culture and Religious Affairs of U.P. Govt. is taking a keen interest in gold plating of the third dome of Temple.

"The frame of the cosmic reality, according to ancient Hindu thought, consists of the three fundamental states called evolution (shrishthi), existence (sthiti), and involution (samhara) that acts in a cyclic process of infinity. Each one of the forms is controlled by Lord Brahma (the creator), Lord Vishnu (the preserver) and Lord Siva/Shiva (the destroyer); these three gods are called the Trinity. Shiva, being the last to complete the cycle from where the new cycle starts, is known as Mahadeo, the Supreme Divinity. The iconographic form of the Shiva, the Linga, represents the unity of the three states of cosmos.

"The Linga consists of the three parts. The first is a square base of three-layers at the bottom showing the three realms, symbolizing evolution, the place of Brahma. The second is an octagonal round form in the middle showing the eight directions, symbolizing existence or perseverance the place of Vishnu, and third is a cylinder at the top with a spherical end, symbolizing involution or completion of the cosmic cycle the place of Shiva. This icon shows the supreme state of integrity, the ultimate form of Shiva linga itself is a symbol of cosmic mandala. As Sadasiva (eternal reality) Shiva is represented as linga, standing also for 'total knowledge.' As Rudra, the destroyer, his consort is Kali. As Bhairava, the terrible destroyer, his consort is Durga. As a jovial god living in the Himalaya, his wife is Parvati. As possessor of all forms of divine power, Shiva rooms at the bottom of everything that is moving; that is how he is called Ishvara, derived from I-cara, i.e., I the center, and cara, the rhythm of movement. Shiva is also depicted as cosmic dancer, Tandava Nartakari, the one who keeps up the rhythm of the world in cosmos.

"Saurashtre Somanathamcha Srisaile Mallikarjunam | Ujjayinya Mahakalam Omkaramamaleswaram | | Paralyam Vaidyanathancha Dakinyam Bheema Shankaram | Setu Bandhethu Ramesam, Nagesam Darukavane | |

"Varanasyantu Vishwesam Tryambakam Gautameethate | Himalayetu Kedaaram, Ghrishnesamcha shivaalaye | | Etani jyotirlingani, Saayam Praatah Patennarah | Sapta Janma Kritam pApam, Smaranena Vinashyati | |

"Mahadev, the Lord, incorporates in Himself the aura and the holiness of all the twelve JyotirLingas. The grandeur of these places is unique and so is their aura. Devotees line up in great numbers to get a holy view of all the Jyotirlingas.

"Location of the Jyotirlinga temples

"Two on the seashore, three on riverbanks, four in the heights of the mountains and three in villages located in meadows; the twelve Jyotirlingas are spread out in a unique and interesting way. Every place has been described in glorious words by many, detailing the surroundings. The story of the origins, and the unique blessings that each one of the sites has to offer.

"Those of us who go to these temples of Shubhankar Shankar-Jyoti-Sivasthan receive the holy blessings of the Lord and come back happy, peaceful and blessed. This indeed depends on one's devotion and experience too.

1. Somnath (Gujarat)
2. Malikarjuna Swami (Andhra Pradesh)
3. Mahakaleshwar (Madhya Pradesh)
4. Omkareshwar (Madhya Pradesh)
5. Kedarnath (Uttarakhand)
6. Bhimashankar (Maharashtra)
7. Kashi Vishwanath Temple (Uttar Pradesh)
8. Trimbakeshwar Shiva Temple (Maharashtra)
9. Nageshvara Jyotirlinga (Gujarat)
10. Baidyanath Temple (Jharkhand)
11. Rameshwar (Tamil Nadu)
12. Grishneshwar (Maharashtra)

It is said that those who chant the Dwadasa Jyotirlinga Stotram, or prayer, will attain salvation and enlightenment and be released from this cycle of human existence with all its travails. By worshipping the Lingas, people of all castes, creeds, and color would be freed from all difficulties. By eating the holy offering made to these Lingas (Naivedyam), one would get rid of all the sins instantly.

"As a matter of fact, we do the Darshan of the JyotirLingas as a part of our daily life. Sun, Fire, and Light, etc., are indeed a part of that great Light. 'Om tatsavituvarenye,' these magical words of the Gayatri mantra, or chant, invoke this Supreme light only. By chanting this powerful Mantra, humans can obtain divine power to their life-light, or Atmajyothi, and seek wisdom and salvation.

"The aura of the sun's rays and the various benefits that can be derived therefrom is indeed a difficult task to describe in words. This gorgeous life-light is the only thing that is responsible for any and every activity in the universe.

'"Agni,' or fire, is a great light. For all the activities on the earth, 'fire' is the pivot.

"Deepajyoti, or light and its greatness, is known to all of us, and we offer our prayers to the holy light. The holy light is offered a place of pride at welcome celebrations and on all auspicious occasions.

"The holy light removes the darkness from the lives of one and all. Darkness means ignorance and it is destroyed by the holy light. The natured light of God makes all our wishes come true when we take a Darshan of it at the Jyotiringas.

"Thus, by taking a Darshan of these twelve Jyotirlingas the auspicious air surrounding them and the holy pilgrimage will bring happiness, peace, and satisfaction to all."

Madhu sat quietly after expressing his idea of the Vishwanath Temple.

I broke the peace that was settling in to the room and said, "Let us understand the prasadam removing sins. Actually, these ancient deities and temples have unique energies in them and the deities are consecrated properly according to Vedic traditions. The milk and food placed on the linga/deities gain that unique positive energy. So, if you eat it, then you gain that unique energy. That helps to reduce the negative energies and actions that you have inside you. That is the meaning of removal of sins. Also, the deities are higher beings in this creation. If we offer prasadam with devotion, it reaches them, and they partake the prasadam from that dimension of the prasadam. At times it is physically eaten also, as I have experienced regularly."

"That is so good to know and understand our ancestors' science behind all rituals and observances," Madhu said with emotion.

The afternoon sun was beating down on us through the drapes on the windows. Madhu decided to leave today as he had to go somewhere.

"I will connect with you soon, Shomikda," he said with a smile before leaving.

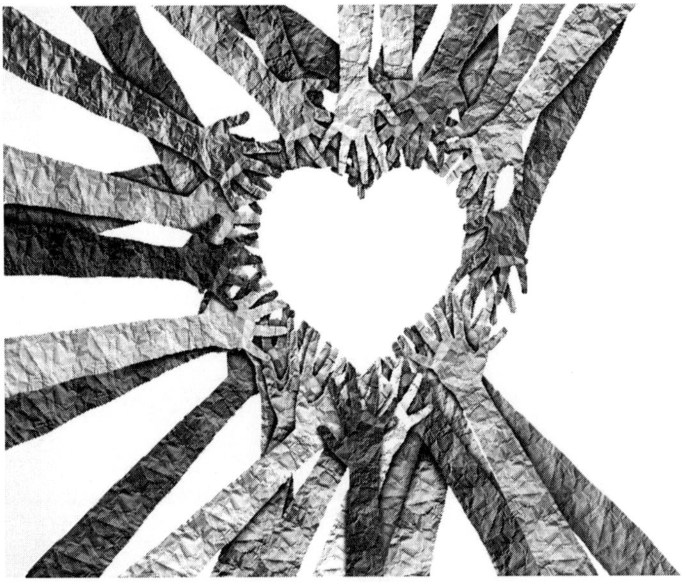

Diverse hands and united diversity or unity partnership in a group of multicultural people globally connected together shaped as a support symbol expressing the feeling of teamwork and togetherness. Credit: wildpixel

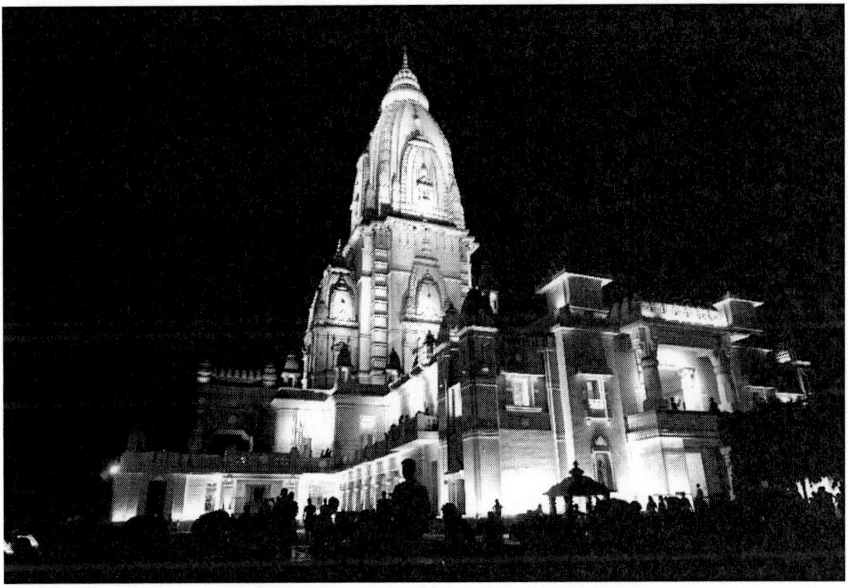

The famous Kashi Vishwanath Temple at Kashi or Varanasi.
Credit: Gaurav Joshi

Chapter 14

Uplifting and Transforming Humanity

It was a Saturday morning when Madhu came to our house. Flurries greeted the holiday season before Christmas by painting a white covering on everything nearby.

My wife had prepared hot coffee along with some snacks that we greedily devoured pretty soon.

Sipping the hot coffee on a cold morning, I began, "Madhu, all this knowledge that I discussed for the past couple of months is from so many teachers, books, sources and Gurus. What is important is to implement that to help humankind and uplift the life on this planet.

"I was honored to be chosen as the youngest United Nations Representative of the UN System in India to the World Summit for Social Development in Copenhagen, Denmark, in March 1995. My specialty was that I focused on human development first than just social development.

"My paper was of the view that social development should start from the lowest level—a human being. For a human being to become better, he has to improve himself physically, mentally, emotionally and spiritually.

"We tend to take care of all the aspects of human existence except spirituality. We must understand, what is spirituality? It is the science of the spirit and the spiritual world. Once we have spirituality as the foundation for our lives, then we are much better human beings, and we are able to bring out the best in us.

"I contended that from the human being, the family gets inspired, from the family the society gets inspired, many such societies create a great nation, and several such nations can create a new world where people look beyond artificial vivisections and embrace the commonalities that we have and live as 'One Earth, One Family.'

"This is a monumental task that needs generations to try and create one. But I believe in slow but steady wins the race. One person, one day at a time, can bring about empowerment. Leaders of the world, both political and social, need to imbibe and inculcate these values. Children should be trained in these values from childhood. The national and local governments need to invest in such training programs for children.

"I was also a cofounder of the NGO Committee on 'Spirituality, Values and Global Concerns' at the United Nations. We endeavored to impress upon the world body on the importance of spirituality in people's lives. It is not about faith, it is about empowering oneself with the infinite, innate, and divine energy that is already there in us.

"I have already written about this energy and its manifestations in earlier chapters. It is not about religion but about empowerment by arousing one's own latent energy. It is called Kula Kundalini, or simply Kundalini.

"Our sages have said for thousands of years about the infinite potentiality of every human being. It is the potential that could take us from the state of a rational animal to the divine state, which is the original and perfect state of existence for all creatures. The door to that state lies at the bottom of our spinal cord and is called Kula Kundalini, an infinite potential energy that is represented as a three-and-a-half coils of a sleeping serpent.

"Kundalini in the form of a 'coiled snake' is a form of divine feminine energy (or Shakti) located at the base of the spine, in the Muladhara chakra. In Śhaiva Tantra, where it is believed to be a force or power associated with the divine feminine or the formless aspect of the goddess. This energy in the body, when cultivated and awakened through spiritual practice, is believed to lead to 'Moksha,' or spiritual liberation. Kuṇḍalinī is associated with Parvati, or Adi Parashakti, the Supreme Being in Shaktism, and with the goddesses Bhairavi and Kubjika. The term, along with practices associated with it, was adopted into Hatha Yoga in the 9th century. It has since then been adopted into other forms of Hinduism as well as modern spirituality and New Age thought.

"Kuṇḍalinī awakenings concentrate on awakening Kuṇḍalinī through meditation, pranayama breathing mainly, and also the practice of asana and chanting of mantras. Kundalini Yoga is influenced by Shaktism and Tantra schools of Hinduism. It derives its name from its focus upon the awakening of Kundalini energy through regular practice of Mantra, Tantra, Yantra, Asanas and Meditation.

"When the Kundalini is aroused, there are two ways of its journey. One is the material movement, which expresses itself in sex. It is wastage of the prized energy. The rishis controlled the physical waste of energy and helped it to rise up the Sushumna, which is a very thin passage or ethereal cord running through spine of the subtle body. This is similar to the spinal cord of the physical body. This vast energy produces frequencies that cannot be produced by our physical bodies or by external energy sources. The subtle nerves get energized and the person can uplift his consciousness from the physical level to a much more elevated level. It is a long and arduous journey filled with pitfalls and distractions. The ultimate state of attainment would take many, many lives and is a journey through one body to the next and next.

"This journey to the spiritual world is considered by the Vedic literature to be a natural journey back home. It also states that only 10 percent of the entire creation is the material world 90 percent constitutes the spiritual world. So, we see how small this infinite material world is in comparison to the actual creation.

"To arouse the Kundalini, we need to follow certain procedures and practices that have been time tested for thousands of years. We also need to follow certain principles like continence, purity, and cleanliness, among others. Most importantly, we have to develop devotion and love of God to attain the highest stages of existence as without that, a sadhaka or person doing penance can easily fall prey to the ego and other pitfalls during the journey.

"This process through meditation is useful not only for the child but also for the family and the community he is associated with.

"Meditation helps a child to inculcate good qualities like concentration, intelligence, forbearance, absence of anger, respect to elders, being creative, and a happy human being spreading love and happiness wherever he/she goes.

"Plus, the most important thing is, he finds a psychological support for himself in the form of God. He also looks at everything with the same eyes as he looks upon himself.

[44]"From children to businesspeople, the values remain the same. In the business arena, a 'radically human organization' is one where leaders are authentic, people are empowered and supported, and everyone feels a sense of purpose, according to Korn Ferry, the human capital consultancy that has popularized the term.

"These progressive organizations understand that a business that focuses only on the 'bottom line' won't enjoy a healthy bottom line for long. They know that sustained success depends upon the people who deliver value and make growth possible.

"They trust that their companies will thrive when, and only if, their people do. Such organizations look at the entire employee experience and embrace doing things differently. They seek less to use people than to support and empower them to do their best work.

"Often, these human-centric organizations are mission-driven (startups are a notable example). Because they value the work that they do in the world, they prize the people that fulfill that mission. For the people who work there, it can become more than just a job.

"Companies like this are vehicles for personal growth and professional development. These organizations care about leaving their employees better than they found them and know that they are better as a result of their employees' involvement. Workplaces that attempt to prioritize business outcomes over the human experience often find that their early successes lack sustainability.

"Radically human organizations have:

- High degree of trust
- Innovation and creativity
- A strong sense of ownership
- People-first approach
- Transparency
- Clear communication
- Authenticity and courage.

"In terms of technology, it can provide the tools for us to grow and change,

[44] *https://www.betterup.com/blog/human-transformation.*

but there's only so much that will happen overnight. It can't, and won't, replace people. We will always rely on each other to contextualize and validate technology-driven change.

"As the world of work becomes increasingly remote and digitally based, it allows us to begin to look at other areas of our lives. When we're not working—when we're not busy adapting to survive—what is it that we need to in order to thrive?

"I would argue that we naturally begin to shift our focus to Inner Transformation to the internal processes that make our outer work more sustainable and more successful. Or, to put it another way, we begin to reach toward self-actualization and human transformation.

"When we understand technology as a tool, we begin to do the real work. That work, in turn, makes us better able to utilize that technology to serve our communities. After all, we are not put on this earth to work indefinitely, but to make it better. That's the real purpose of our lives, our work, and of our inner transformation.

[45]"The World Humanitarian Summit (Istanbul, May 2016) was a pivotal moment for the global community toward human empowerment through ensuring basic needs. It generated momentum and political determination to move forward on the Agenda for Humanity and its five core responsibilities, and kickstarted concrete changes in the way we address humanitarian need, risk and vulnerability.

"At the Summit, nine thousand participants representing 180 Member States of the United Nations, over seven hundred local and international NGOs, the private sector and other stakeholders demonstrated overwhelming support for the transformations called for in the Agenda for Humanity.

"This support is evidenced by the nearly three thousand commitments to action, and over 2,500 alignments with the core commitments and nearly twenty initiatives and partnerships that were launched to deliver the changes that are needed.

"Now the hard work of delivering these transformations and making lasting improvements for people caught up in crises begins.

---

[45] *https://www.unocha.org/about-us/agenda-humanity.*

"The Agenda for Humanity

- Political leadership to prevent and end conflicts
- Uphold norms that safeguard humanity
- Leave no one behind
- Change people's lives from delivering aid to ending need
- Invest in humanity

"The world is at a critical juncture. Some 132 million people around the world are in urgent need of humanitarian assistance and protection—the highest numbers since the Second World War. Millions more are affected by fragility, conflicts and vulnerability. This is why former Secretary-General Ban Ki-moon put forward a new Agenda for Humanity, calling on global leaders to stand up for our common humanity and reduce humanitarian suffering.

"The Agenda consists of five Core Responsibilities and twenty-four transformations that are needed to achieve progress to address and reduce humanitarian need, risk and vulnerability. Together, they form a framework for action, change and mutual accountability against which we can collectively assess and review progress in order to reduce the suffering of millions of people, and address and reduce humanitarian need, risk and vulnerability.

"Such endeavors can help reduce poverty and helplessness and uplift people from the trenches to a decent living.

"To me leadership is very important as they sign on the future of a nation of people. So good leaders must be given positions of power and responsibility to fulfill their responsibility toward humanity.

"But it is wrong to leave everything to the leaders and expect them to work miracles. Development is from the top, the bottom and from the middle. People from the grassroot level and other levels must coordinate to bring empowerment and development in every strata of the society. Then only would true, sustainable and all-encompassing development take place."

Madhu stared at me for some time and finally said, "Shomikda, you seem to have a solution for all problems."

"No, I do not, my friend. But I believe that advancement in spirituality and evolution of consciousness enhance the happiness from within and also enable a human being to fulfill his duties and responsibilities much better. Human upliftment and transformation can take place only through the evolution of consciousness," I replied with a little embarrassment.

Madhu started on his experience lecture. "Shomikda, I visited the Badrinath temple and it was a wonderful experience of history, structure and importance.

"As you know, [46]Badrinath, or Badrinarayana, Temple is a temple dedicated to Lord Vishnu. It is situated in the town of Badrinath in Uttarakhand, India. The temple is also one of the 108 Divya Desams dedicated to Vishnu—holy shrines for Vaishnavas—who is worshipped as Badrinath. It is open for six months every year (between the end of April and the beginning of November), because of extreme weather conditions in the Himalayan region. The temple is located in Garhwal hill tracks in Chamoli district along the banks of Alakananda River. It is one of the most visited pilgrimage centers of India, having recorded 2.8 million visits in just two months in 2022. It is one of the Char Dham pilgrimage sites.

"The image of the presiding deity worshipped in the temple is a 1-foot-(0.30-meter)black granite deity of Vishnu in the form of Badrinarayan. The deity is considered by many Hindus to be one of eight *svayam vyakta kshetras*, or self-manifested deities of Vishnu.

"Mata Murti Ka Mela, which commemorates the descent of River Ganges on Mother Earth, is the most prominent festival celebrated in the Badrinath Temple. Although Badrinath is located in North India, the head priest, or Rawal, is traditionally a Nambudiri Brahmin chosen from the South Indian state of Kerala. The temple was included in the Uttar Pradesh state government Act, which later came to be known as Shri Badarinath and Shri Kedarnath Mandir Act. The committee nominated by the state government administers both the temples and has seventeen members on its board.

"The temple is mentioned in ancient religious texts like *Vishnu Purana* and *Skanda Purana*. It is glorified in the *Naalayira Divya Prabandham*, an early medieval Tamil canon of the Alvar saints from the 6th–9th centuries C.E.

"Adi Shankara established Badrinath as a pilgrimage site in the ninth century. The temple has three structures: the Garbhagriha (sanctum), the Darshan Mandapa (worship hall), and Sabha Mandapa (convention hall). The conical-shaped roof of the sanctum, the *garbhagriha*, is approximately 15 meters (49 feet) tall with a small cupola on top, covered with a gold gilt roof. The facade is built of stone and has arched windows. A broad stairway leads up to the main entrance, a tall arched gateway. Just inside is a mandap, a large pillared hall

[46] *Incredibleindia.org.*

that leads to the sanctum, or main shrine area. The walls and pillars of the hall are covered with intricate carvings.

"The main shrine houses the 1-foot-(0.30-meter) Shaligram (black stone) deity of Badrinarayana, which is housed in a gold canopy under a Badri Tree. The deity of Badrinarayana shows Him holding a *Shankha* (conch) and a *Chakra* (wheel) in two of His arms in a lifted posture and the other two arms resting on His lap in a *Yogamudra* (*Padmasana*) posture. The sanctum also houses images of the god of wealth—Kubera, sage Narada, Uddhava, Nara and Narayana. There are fifteen more images that are also worshipped around the temple. These include that of Lakshmi, Garuda (the vahana of Narayan), and Navadurga, the manifestation of Durga in nine different forms. The temple also has shrines of Lakshmi Narasimhar and for saints Adi Shankara (C.E. 788-820), Nar and Narayan, Ghantakarna, Vedanta Desika and Ramanujacharya. All the deities of the temple are made of black stone.

"The Tapt Kund, a group of hot Sulphur springs just below the temple, is considered to be medicinal; many pilgrims consider it a requirement to bathe in the springs before visiting the temple. The springs have a year-round temperature of 55°C (131°F), while outside temperature is typically below 17°C (63°F) all year 'round. The two water ponds in the temple are called Narad Kund and Surya Kund.

"There is no historical record about the temple, but there is a mention of the presiding deity Badrinath in Vedic scriptures. According to some accounts, the shrine was worshipped in some form in the Vedic period. The architecture of the temple resembling that of a Buddhist vihara (temple) and the brightly painted façade, which is atypical of Buddhist temples, leads to the argument. Other accounts relate that it was originally established as a pilgrimage site by Adi Shankara in the ninth century. It is believed that Shankara resided in the place for six years, from C.E. 814 to 820. He resided six months in Badrinath and the rest of the year in Kedarnath. Hindu followers assert that he discovered the deity of Badrinath in the Alaknanda River and enshrined it in a cave near the Tapt Kund hot springs. A traditional story asserts that Shankara expelled all the Buddhists in the region with the help of the Parmar ruler King Kanak Pal; however, this might be fictitious and very recent. The hereditary successors of the king governed the temple and endowed villages to meet its expenses. The income from a set of villages on the route to the temple was used to feed and accommodate pilgrims. The Parmar rulers held the title 'Bolanda Badrinath,' meaning speaking Badrinath. They had other titles, including Shri 108 Basdrishcharyaparayan Garharaj Mahimahendra, Dharmabibhab, and Dharamarakshak Sigamani.

"The throne of Badrinath was named after the presiding deity; the king enjoyed ritual obeisance by the devotees before proceeding to the shrine. The practice was continued until the late 19th century. During the 16th century, the king of Garhwal moved the murti to the present temple. When the state of Garhwal was divided, the Badrinath temple came under British rule but the king of Garhwal continued as the chairman of the management committee. The selection of priest is done after consultation between Garhwal and Travancore royal families.

"The temple has undergone several major renovations due to its age and damage by an avalanche. In the 17th century, the temple was expanded by the kings of Garhwal. After significant damage during the great 1803 Garhwal earthquake, it was largely rebuilt by the king of Jaipur. It was still under renovation as late as the 1870s but these were completed by the time of the First World War. At that time, the town was still small, consisting of only the twenty-odd huts housing the temple's staff, but the number of pilgrims was usually between seven and ten thousand. The Kumbha Mela festival, held every twelve years, raised the number of visitors to fifty thousand. The temple also enjoyed revenue from the rents owed to it by various villages bequeathed by various rajas."

Madhu stopped, pleased with his description as I nodded and smiled in appreciation during his talk.

After some less important talk, he proceeded to leave for the day.

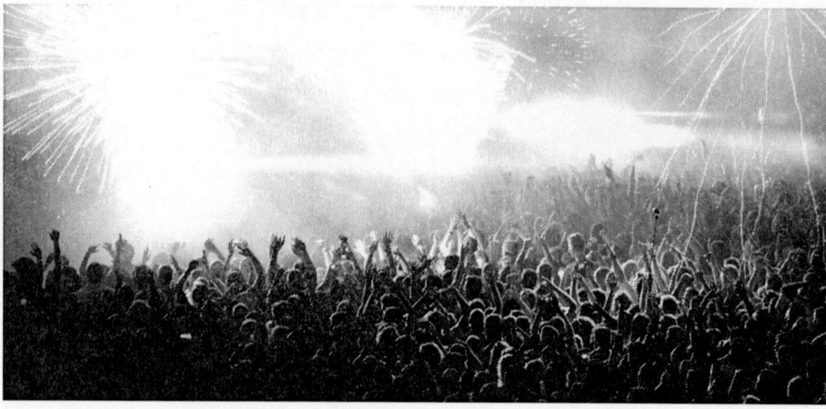

Bringing humanity to the light of Godhead.
Credit: 8213erika

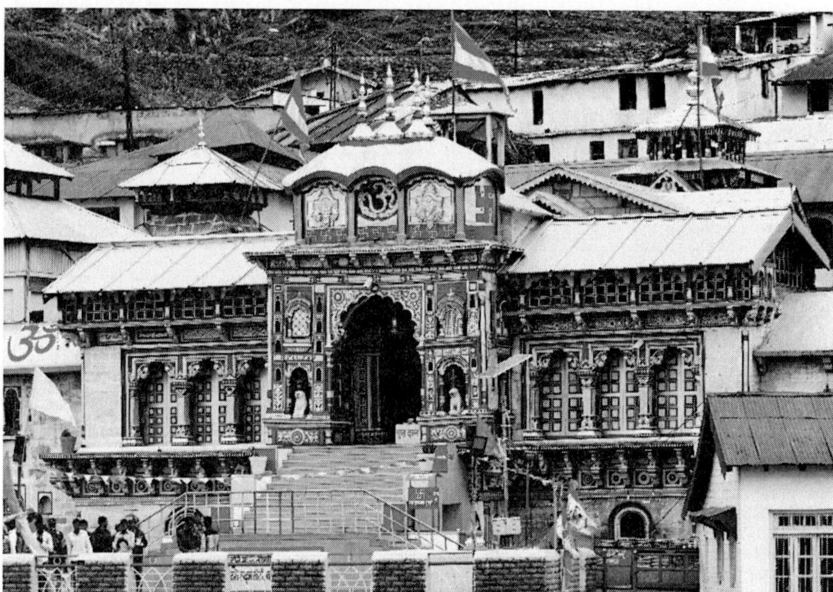

The famous Badrinath Temple in Uttarakhand.
Credit: Sujithkumar VD

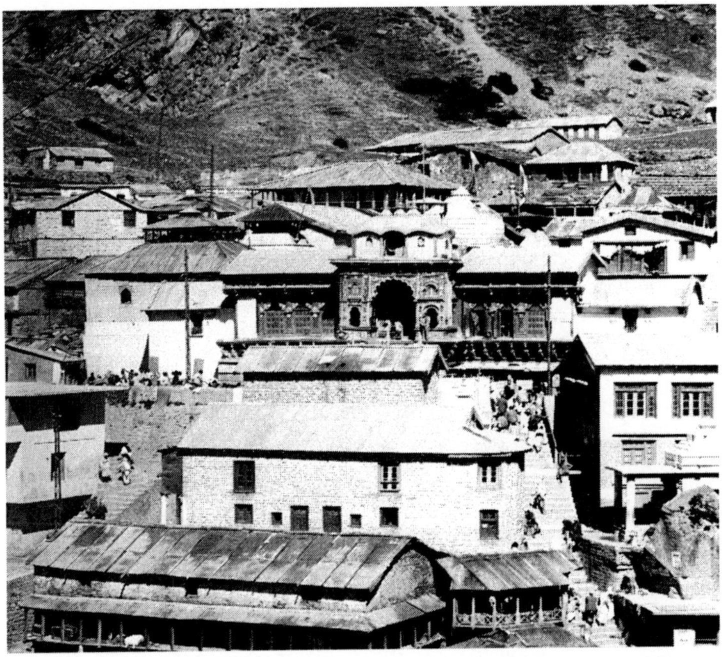

Badrinath Temple. Credit: Ministry of External Affairs, Government of India

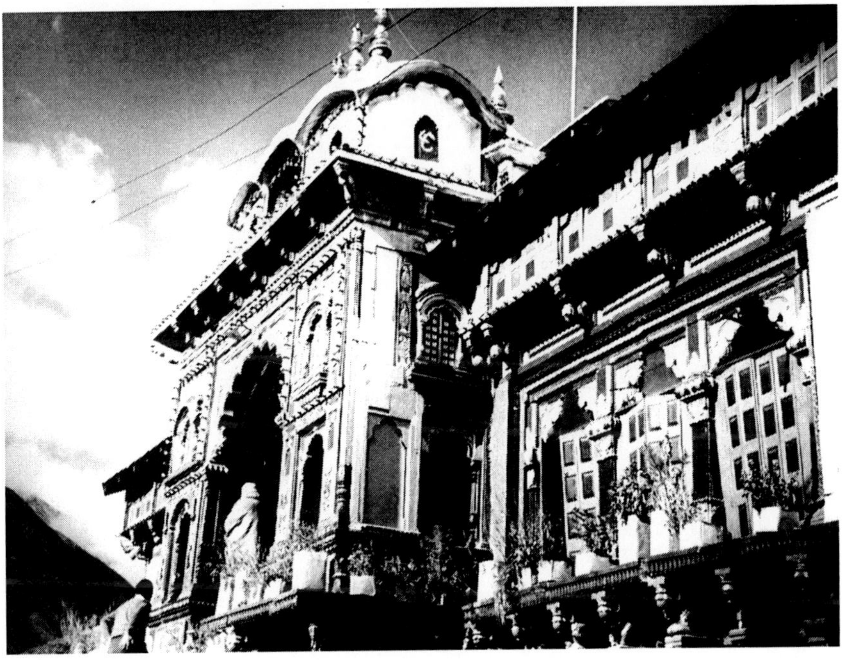

Badrinath Temple. Credit: Ministry of External Affairs, Government of India

Chapter 15

Ushering In the Golden Age for Humankind

Madhu was early on Sunday morning. "Shomikda, I cannot wait to hear more from you. I came here early today. I hope you don't mind," he said while settling into the sofa.

"Of course, it is our pleasure to have you today or at any time. It is our pleasure and privilege to have you," I answered, joining him on the sofa.

Coffee was served hot by my dear wife again.

"Today I will talk about the result of all these austerities that I have talked about earlier. It will help bring in a golden age for the planet.

"Historians refer to certain time periods of some civilizations as golden ages. Golden ages are periods of great wealth, prosperity, stability, and cultural and scientific achievement.

"Human existence in this world has undergone a series of ages. As one of the greatest ages for humanity, the golden age represents the first period of human existence, when humans flourished in various aspects.

"Humans lived superb lives during the golden age because they enjoyed peace, coexisted in harmony, depended on stable governments, and attained significant prosperity. However, the emergence of new philosophies, ideologies, religious doctrines, and cultural norms brought the golden age to an end and ushered in subsequent human eras.

"Let us now understand the Yuga system of time calculation in the Hindu or Indian system.

[47]"In the yogic astronomy, we divide the orbit of the Earth around the Sun

[47] *IshaFoundation.org.*

into twenty-seven segments, called nakshatras. Each nakshatra is further divided into four equal sectors called padas, or steps. Multiply four by twenty-seven and it equals 108. These 108 units mark the 108 steps that the Earth takes through space. Each nakshatra corresponds to one half of the lunar orbit around the Earth. The cycles within the human body respond and correspond to that.

"The Nakshatras and Padas

"In a woman's body, there are very obvious cycles of 27.55 days if she is perfectly healthy. In a man's body, the cycles are less obvious and pronounced – they happen in a different way and are of a larger span of time. In any case, these cycles are happening all the time in the solar system and the larger universe. The microcosm and the macrocosm both are playing the same game. But who should play whose game? If you think the macrocosm is going to play your game, you will waste your life. If you play the macrocosm's game, your life will be beyond your expectations.

"The Cycle of Four Yugas

"The precession (caused by gradual rotation of the Earth's axis) of the Equinoxes is the period of time that it takes the Earth's axis to pass through one complete cycle of the zodiac. It takes the planet 72 years to go through one degree of the zodiac and 25,920 years to complete one full circle of 360 degrees. One half of the journey takes 12,960 years and covers the four Yugas. Satya Yuga lasts 5184 years. Treta Yuga lasts 3888 years. Dwapara Yuga lasts 2592 years. Kali Yuga lasts 1296 years. These four Yugas taken together come to a total of 12,960 years.

"When did Kali Yuga start?

"The story of Mahabharata needs to be seen in a certain context. In about 3140 B.C. the Kurukshetra War ended, and about thirty-five years after that Lord Krishna left his body. Kali Yuga started after that. As of 2023 Krishna's era ended 5128 years ago. If you subtract 2592, which is the cumulative number of years of the two Kali Yugas that are at the bottom of the ellipse, which describes the axial precession, you arrive at 2536 years. That means we have already completed 2536 years of Dwapara Yuga, and since its total duration is 2592 years, we still have fifty-six years until its completion. In the year 2079, we will complete Dwapara Yuga and move on to Treta Yuga. The world will go through another upheaval, not necessarily in terms of war but probably in terms of population explosion and natural calamities, before moving on to this new era of wellbeing and upward movement of human consciousness.

"Yugas and Human Consciousness

"The solar system with the sun and the planets around it is moving in the galaxy. It takes 25,920 years for our solar system to complete one cycle around a larger star. From the effects upon the planet, we believe this big star or big system that our system is going around is not located in the center of the orbit but somewhere to the side. Whenever our solar system comes closer to this big system, all the creatures living in our system rise to greater possibilities. Whenever our system moves away from it, the creatures living in our system come to the lowest level of possibility— we say this is Kali Yuga.

"When our solar system is closer to the 'Super Sun,' Satya Yuga will begin. The human mind will be at its highest competence. People's ability to know life, people's ability to communicate, people's ability to live happily will be at its highest. In other words, we will have levelheaded people, all it takes to live well on this planet is a bunch of levelheaded people.

"In Satya Yuga, human ability to communicate will be at its best because the ether will be very close. Right now, the etheric sphere of the planet is raised to a certain point. There was a time when it was much higher—now it has come a little closer. [48]When the ether is very close and I want to convey something to you, I do not have to say it. Even when my eyes are closed, you will know what I want to say. When the ether rises a little bit but is still at a certain distance, if I close my eyes, you will not know, but if I open my eyes and look at you, you will know what I want to convey.

"At the same time, no matter which time, which yuga, which planetary position we are in right now, still individual human beings can rise above all this. Still individual human beings can live in a golden time within themselves. Even in the worst of times, the possibility to be well above it is always there for a human being.

"There are many things one can do to enhance the ether or create etheric content. This is why Lord Krishna said, in Kali Yuga, which is down there, far

[48] Four stages of speech: Para, which finds manifestation only in Prana; Pasyanti, which finds manifestation in the mind; Madhyama, which finds manifestation in the Indriyas; and Vaikhari, which finds manifestation in articulate expression.

away from the Super Sun, the ether will be so low that there is no point in trying to teach them Yoga, meditation, mantras or yantras—they will not get it. Just teach them devotion. If they are devout, they will generate their own ether. And because of this etheric content in the atmosphere, they will perceive. Devotion is not for the dumb—but even if you are the dumbest, you can still get it.

"Thousands of years ago, they said that as the solar system moves closer to the Super Sun, human intelligence will blossom. As the solar system moves closer, the realization that the whole body and the whole universe are electric structures will come naturally.

"Lord Krishna also said that after over five thousand years, there will come a many-thousand-year period of time that will be fabulous. We will not make it there, but we can set the foundations for it for succeeding generations for a period for thousands of years a golden age on earth.

"This is not all prediction and conjecture, this based on a deep-rooted understanding about what happens with the human mind in relation to the planet on which you live. We do not live on this planet. We are the planet. If you do not understand this today, you will understand when you die that we go back to the earth from which we came.

"The preparation for this golden age means that we have to practice and uplift our consciousness above the regular material objects only to the higher level of existence. Then only the qualities that are required for a golden age or a harmonious society will evolve. So, if we encourage people to follow the path of devotion along with Yoga, OM Kriya Yoga, mantra chanting and prepare under guidance of the Yoga Sutras of Patanjali, the world can expect the Golden Age or era to be ushered in over the next generation or two."

I sat back with my coffee and looked at Madhu. He was overwhelmed and looked with deep interest.

"So, there is light at the end of the tunnel out of this global mess that humankind has created?" he questioned.

"Yes, there is. That is part of the civilizational and Yuga cycle," I answered. "Tell me about your visit to Dwarakadish Temple of Gujarat. I believe you had visited that temple?" I asked.

"Yes, Shomikda," he said, "I visited the temple in Gujarat.[49]The Dwarkadhish temple, also known as the Jagat Mandir, is a temple dedicated to

---

[49] *Incredibleindia.org.*

Lord Krishna, who is worshiped here by the name *Dwarkadhish*, or 'King of Dwarka.' The temple is located at Dwarka city of Gujarat, India, which is one of the destinations of Char Dham (four holy pilgrimage places), a Hindu pilgrimage circuit. The main shrine of the five-storied building, supported by seventy-two pillars, is known as Jagat Mandir, or Nija Mandir. Archaeological findings suggest the original temple was built in 200 B.C.E. at the earliest. The temple was rebuilt and enlarged in the 15th-16th century. According to tradition, the original temple was believed to have been built by Krishna's grandson, Vajranabha, over the harigriha (Krishna's residential place). The original structure was destroyed by Mahmud Begada in 1472 and subsequently rebuilt in the 15th-16th century in the Mru-Gurjara style.

"The temple became part of the *Char Dham* pilgrimage considered sacred by Hindus in India. Adi Shankaracharya, the 8th Century saint and philosopher, visited the shrine. The other three being comprising Rameswaram, Badrinath and Puri. Even today a memorial within the temple is dedicated to his visit. Dwarakadheesh is the 98th Divya Desam of Vishnu on the subcontinent, glorified in the *Divya Prabandha* sacred texts. The temple is at an elevation of 12.19 meters (40.0 feet) above mean sea-level. It faces west. The temple layout consists of a garbhagriha (*Nijamandira* or *Harigraha*) and an antarala (an antechamber). However, the existing temple is dated to 16th century.

"The current temple in Chaulukya style was constructed in the 15th-16th centuries. The temple covers an area of 27 meters by 21 meters with east-west length of 29 meters and north-south width of 23 meters. The tallest peak of the temple is 51.8 meters high.

"Since this site is associated with the ancient city of Dwaraka and Lord Krishna of Mahabharata times, it is an important place of pilgrimage for Hindus. It is one of three main pilgrimage sites related to *'Krishna'* circuit, namely *48 kos parikrama of Kurukshetra* in Haryana state, Braj Parikarma in Mathura of Uttar Pradesh state and *Dwarka Parikrama* (Dwarkadish Yatra) at Dwarkadhish Temple in Gujarat state.

"The flag atop the temple shows the sun and moon, which is believed to indicate that Lord Krishna would be there till the sun and moon exist on Earth. The flag is changed up to five times a day, but the symbol remains the same. The temple has a five-story structure built on seventy-two pillars. The temple spire is 78.3 meters high. The temple is constructed of limestone, which is still in pristine condition. The temple shows intricate sculptural detailing.

"There are two entrances to the temple. The main entrance (north entrance) is called 'Moksha Dwara' (Door to Salvation). This entrance takes one to the main market. The south entrance is called 'Swarga Dwara' (Gate to Heaven). Outside this doorway are fifty-six steps that lead to the Gomati River. Though the origins are not clearly known, the Advaita School of Hinduism, established by Sankaracharya, who created Hindu monastic institutions across India, attributes the origin of Char Dham to the seer. The four monasteries are located across the four corners of India and their attendant temples are Badrinath Temple at Badrinath in the North, Jagannath Temple at Puri in the East, Dwarakadheesh Temple at Dwarka in the West and Ramanathaswamy Temple at Rameswaram in the South. Though ideologically the temples are divided between the sects of Hinduism, namely Saivism and Vaishnavism, the Char Dham pilgrimage is an all-Hindu affair. There are four abodes in Himalayas called Chota Char Dham (*Chota* meaning small): Badrinath, Kedarnath, Gangotri and Yamunotri—all these lie at the foothills of Himalayas. The name *Chota* was added during the mid-20th century to differentiate the original Char Dhams. As the number of pilgrims increased to these places in modern times, it is called Himalayan Char Dham. The journey across the four cardinal points in India is considered sacred by Hindus, who aspire to visit these temples once in their lifetime. Traditionally the trip starts are the eastern end from Puri, proceeding in clockwise direction in a manner typically followed for circumambulation in Hindu temples. The Krishna Janmashtami festival, or Gokulashtami, the birthday of Krishna, was commissioned by Vallaba (1473-1531).

"According to a legend, Meera Bai, the famed Rajput princess who was also a poetess-saint and a staunch devotee of Krishna, merged with the deity at this temple. It is one of the Sapta Puri, the seven holy cities of India.

"The temple is also the location of Dvaraka Pitha, one of the four *peeths* (religious centers) established by Adi Shankaracharya (686-717), who pioneered unification of Hindu religious beliefs in the country. It is a four-storied structure representing four *peeths* established by Shankaracharya in different parts of the country. There are paintings on the walls here depicting the life history of Shankaracharya while the dome has carvings of Shiva in different postures.

"It is a five-storied edifice built over seventy-two pillars (sandstone temple with sixty pillars is also mentioned). There are two important entrances to the temple, one is the main entry door, which is called the *Moksha Dwar* (meaning 'Door to Salvation'), and the exit door, which is known as the *Swarga Dwar* (meaning 'Gate to Heaven').

"The main deity deified in the sanctum is of Dwarkadeesh, which is known as Trivikrama form of Vishnu and is depicted with four arms. On the chamber to the left of the main altar is the deity of Balarama, elder brother of Krishna. The chamber to the right houses the images of Pradyumna and Aniruddha, son and grandson of Krishna. In several shrines surrounding the central shrine there are idols of goddess Radha, Jambavati, Satyabhama and Lakshmi. Shrines of Madhav Raoji (another name for Krishna), Balarama and sage Durvasa are also present in the temple. There are also two separate shrines dedicated to Radha Krishna and Devaki just in front of the central shrine of Dwarkadhish.

"Carvings around the platform

"The temple spire rises to a height of 78 meters (256 feet) and a very large flag with symbols of the sun and moon is hoisted on it. The flag, triangular in shape, is 50 feet (15 meters) length. This flag is changed four times a day with a new one and Hindus pay a huge sum of money to hoist it by purchasing a new flag. The money received on this account is credited to the trust fund of the temple to meet the operation and maintenance expenses of the temple."

"Shomikda, I feel blessed to visit so many ancient temples of India, which are exquisite in their architecture and divine in their ambience. The entire ecosystems of these temples are so uplifting and divine. You gain a lot of positive energy by simply going there and absorbing the energy. I still do not have a family. Then these journeys would not have happened to the extent that it has happened now. But I do not miss a family. These temples and people like you are my family," was an emotional outburst from Madhu.

"Madhu, my dear friend, we are indeed your family. You are part of our family. For the past few months we have discussed so much about spirituality, your visits to temples and the rejuvenation and upliftment of humanity. Now comes the time to reach out to the multitude to read all this in the form of a book. Let us hope this book will see the dawn of day someday by God's grace," I said as I ended the talk for the day for lunch.

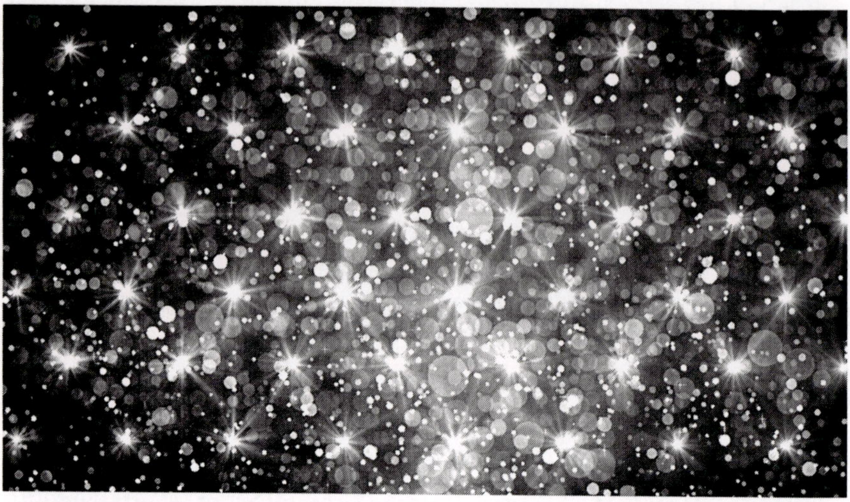

Artistic depiction of a Golden Age. Credit: urzine

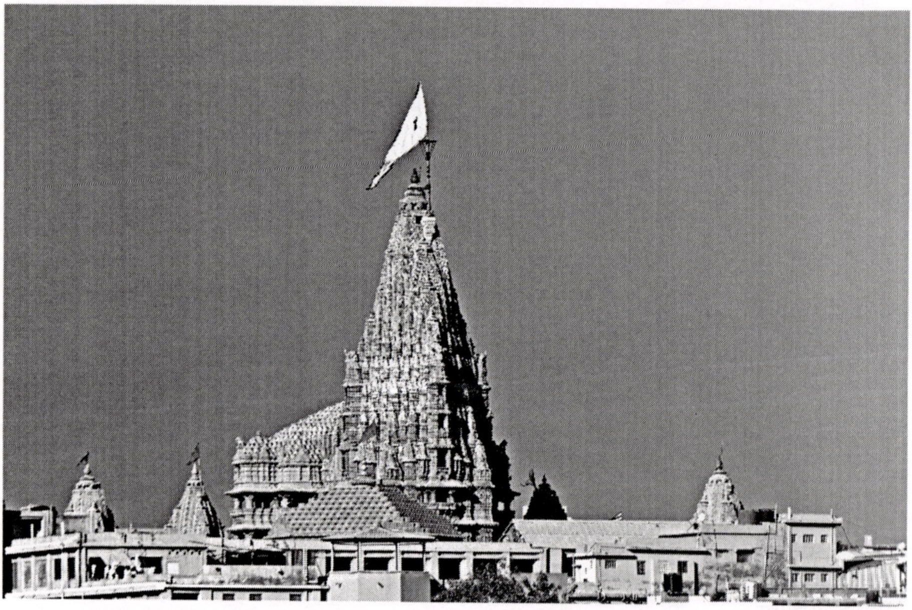

Ancient and famous temple of Shri Krishna Dwarakadish, Dwaraka City, Gujarat. Credit: vbel71